How to **STAY HEALTHY**

and still **Eat CHOCOLATE**

How to STAY HEALTHY and still Eat CHOCOLATE

The essential guide to creating a
healthy home environment, diet, and lifestyle.

Karen Alison with Kathy Raymond

Artemis House
Barrie, Canada

Illustrations: Copyright King Features Syndicate. Reprinted with permission-The Toronto Star Syndicate

Cover Design: Brian Cartwright, Rocket Design
Text Design: Jessica Burton
Printed in Canada by Transcontinental

National Library of Canada Cataloguing in Publication Data
Alison, Karen.
    How to stay healthy and still eat chocolate.

Includes bibliographical references and index.
ISBN 0-9688704-0-6

    1. Health. I. Raymond, Kathy. II. Title.

RA776.A552001   613   C2001-900855-4

The following trademarks appear in the text: Almay, Aveda "All Sensitive", Ancient Harvest, Avalon Organics, Bach Rescue Remedy, Baker's Mate, Bionaire, Burt's Bees, Clinique, Cool Hemp, Corningware, Earthwise, Ecosave, Ecover, Edenblend, Frontier, Gaiam, Greens+, Herbal Glo, Karitea, Keri Lotion, Kettle Valley, Kyo-dophilus, Lubriderm, Marcelle, Mum's, Natracare, Natural Dentist Herbal Mouth and Gum Therapy, Nature Clean, Nature's Blends, Nature's Gate, Nu-Life Dyna-Gest Ultra-Zyme, Nutra Sprout, Olbas, Ombrelle, Organic Essentials, Orange aPEEL, Peelu, Prairie Naturals, President's Choice, Pure Synergy, Pyrex, Raja's Cup, Rapidura, Ray Away, Rice Dream, Soap Factory, Soy Delicious, Sucanat, Sweet Nothings, Swiss Herbal, Tampax, The Body Shop, The Missing Link, Udo's Choice, Unpetroleum, Webber, Weleda, Wobenzym.

Note: All products mentioned throughout the book are proprietary to their manufacturers or creators, whether or not the symbols ™ or ® accompany product or company names.

10 9 8 7 6 5 4 3 2 1

This book is dedicated to Sherry, Jon, and Jake.
And to our home, Earth.

Acknowledgments:

Many people have generously contributed time, love, expertise, and encouragement to this project. The authors gratefully acknowledge the following for assistance, support, feedback, suggestions, information, enthusiasm, and the loan of the table: (in alphabetical order) Gordon Alison, Adrienne Alison, the Almeidas, Marcellus Anderson, Liz Antonacci, Dawn Bell, Jonathan van Bilsen, Dan Bodanis, Paul Bonish, Maureen Borghoff, Theo Colborn, Ted Cowan, Paola DeMaria, Mike Ellis, Udo Erasmus, Lorraine Flanigan, Elaine Gottschall, Rob Grand and Grassroots, everyone at Harmony Market, Karen Hawes, Inkwe, Gwen Perlman King, Diane & John Lightowler, Taivi Lobu, Cathy McCartney, Misha, Faith Moffatt, Jon & Jake Oelrichs, Miriam Owen, Sheila Pennington, Dennis Robitaille, Hilary Rowland, Liivi Ruona, Michael Sachter, Bonnie Service, Tilda Shalof, Cheryl Shour, Brenda Spencer, Barb Taylor, the Toronto Environmental Alliance, Sana Valliani, and Susan Williamson. If we have left anyone out, we apologize profusely. Thanks, everyone! We couldn't have done it without you.

Special thanks to Gordon Alison, Dawn Bell, Paola Demaria, and Mike Ellis. You know why.

About the authors

Karen Alison (right) dates her fascination with natural wellness to the age of 14, when the first health food store in her neighbourhood opened its doors. Her mother encouraged her curiosity by dismissing all wellness practitioners and health food store owners as quacks. Karen has been exploring and researching the many modalities of natural health and nutrition ever since.

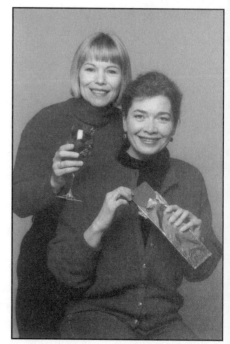

Karen graduated from Queen's University, and has taken certificates in Working with Adult Children and Codependents, and coaching Life Skills. Among the healing techniques she has studied are reiki, massage therapy, Therapeutic Touch, Touch for Health, energy balancing and sensitivity testing with acupressure and applied kinesiology, macrobiotics, addictive nutrition, and five-phase nutrition.

She lives with one man, two dogs, and a cat.

Kathy Raymond (left) runs a private practice where she uses Applied Kinesiology to assess sensitivities. Kathy has a B.A. in psychology from Queen's University and is certified by the International Kinesiology College as a Touch for Health instructor. She provides workshops which lead to certification in all four levels of Touch for Health.

Kathy is available for lectures and classes in various aspects of natural wellness and nutrition. For more information, contact her through Artemis House, P.O. Box 1449, Barrie, Ontario, L4M 5R4. (Also see the order form at the end of this book.)

Contents

HOW IT ALL BEGAN...

At four o'clock in the morning on February 12, the phone rang. Even before I picked it up, I knew what it meant. I knew my mother had died.

We rushed through the freezing night to the hospital. As our family gathered around my mother's bed for the last time, shock and sorrow filled the room. At the same time, I sensed a feeling of relief that my mother's pain and suffering were over. Her two-year struggle with bone cancer had been ugly and terrible, and the treatments for it seemed equally cruel. Yet right up until a few weeks before her death, my mother had continued her architectural work, building a house for my father and herself. Now she would not live in it. She would not see her grandchildren grow up, continue her intellectual pursuits, or visit with her large, interesting circle of friends. She was 68 years old. I looked at my mother's still form and wondered, *Did it have to happen like this?*

In the days that followed, I returned to this question and one other many times. The second question was even more frightening. *Will this happen to me?*

I looked at other members of our family for clues. No one else had died of cancer, and most of the older members were long-lived. Yet many of them shared health complaints: arthritis, high blood pressure, digestive trouble, and various other chronic conditions. Then I looked at my own state of health. When I started to pay attention, I realized I had joint pain, no energy, food cravings, swelling and tingling in my hands, cold hands and feet even on the warmest day, thinning hair, constant indigestion, roller coaster emotions, and my nose ran all the time even when I didn't have a cold! I often felt like a tired 150-year-old.

Was this normal? Or were these some kind of signals I didn't know how to read? What would happen if I ignored them and went on with my typical North American lifestyle? I was only in my 30's. What kind of signals would I get in another 10 or 20 years? What condition would I be in by the time *I* was 68?

I had a choice to make. I could leave everything to chance or I could learn how to read the signals and find out what, if anything, I could do about them. I chose to learn.

The first thing I learned was that my doctor, while excellent at working with sick people, had no advice for me. I was not actually ill or in a crisis state, and she had been trained to work with physical trauma and disease. Since I had no idea how to find a doctor who could help me, I moved on to wellness professionals, people who would teach me how to be healthy and stay that way.*

From them, I learned that my symptoms were definite signals about my state of health. And those signals *all* meant something, in the present and for the future. I could ignore them at my peril!

I didn't want to ignore them. For one thing, having seen some possible consequences, I was scared. But more than that, I was intrigued. What would it feel like to get rid of all these annoying and sometimes embarrassing symptoms? What were the possibilities in life for someone who felt really good all the time? What would I have to do to find myself ahead of the health game instead of always playing catch-up? How might my future open up if I could grow older without the arthritis and other chronic degenerative conditions I saw in family members?

*At the time, the practice of clinical ecology, or environmental medicine, was illegal where I lived. In this speciality, doctors look at the larger picture affecting the health of the individual, rather than focussing on individual symptoms or organs, and include healing techniques complementary to allopathic medicine.

I was excited by the possibilities. I explored health techniques with a wide range of teachers, read everything I could about health and healing, and visited healers and wellness practitioners for treatments. A few of these people seemed a bit flaky to me. But most had solid, practical information or services to offer, based on years of education and working with clients. I began to put together the best of the knowledge I received and apply it in my life.

At first, my friends and family had mixed reactions to my experiments on myself. Some were hostile, others called me a "nut". I realized they were giving me the same treatment Thomas Edison got a century ago for his idea of creating an electric lightbulb. People thought he was crazy. Now, it's hard to imagine life *without* the lightbulb. Encouraged by this thought, I got together with some other "nuts" and we motivated each other to keep learning.

The first thing I learned was that my body could and would heal itself, if I gave it the support and encouragement it needed. Then I learned that I didn't have to get sick and fall apart as I got older. I began to find answers to my questions, including the two I asked after my mother died. I discovered how simple but powerful choices could improve my current health and prevent future problems.

Making these choices was like gaining a new life. Over time all my symptoms disappeared, my health improved dramatically, and I began to feel much younger than my chronological age. I grew more confident and enjoyed my life as I hadn't since childhood. My weight stabilized. I found I had more available time, because I was no longer losing hours to fatigue and recuperation from ailments. Best of all, I found out I didn't have to give up everything I enjoyed. I could stay healthy and still eat chocolate!

People began to notice. After a while, many began to ask me how *they* could make similar improvements in their own lives. They didn't want to read dozens of books and articles or visit every wellness practitioner in town. They didn't want to quit drinking coffee or eat only bean sprouts and tofu. They *did* want to know the simple, practical steps they could take to improve their well-being right away and for the long-term.

This book is written for them and for you. I hope it brings you answers to some of your own questions. It is packed with health-maximizing ideas from over a decade of study and client work to help you make informed choices. When you make these choices, you give yourself power: the power to enjoy good health for your whole life! And still eat chocolate.

TO BEGIN WITH...

The information in this chapter is not intended as a replacement for medical care or the advice of a physician. In the case of any illness or trauma, seek medical assistance immediately.

1. BASICS. YOUR IMMUNE SYSTEM AND TOTAL TOXIC LOAD.

Do you think of good health as a matter of becoming perfect and then staying that way for the rest of your life? Perfection is too much of a challenge for me. Instead, I think of health as a journey where you make many little shifts in direction over time, similar to the way you would navigate a boat. A few small course corrections can make a huge difference in your eventual destination.

Most of this book details the many shifts in direction—or steps—you can take to improve your health. Each chapter covers a specific topic. The steps look simple but when you combine them, you can create major positive results, the kind of results that let you stay healthy and still eat chocolate.

As you read through this book, you may find yourself resisting some of the information in it. That's okay! While both of us have done pretty much everything we've written about in the following chapters, our progress wasn't always straightforward.

Some of the steps were easy and quick. Others took much longer and were more challenging, largely because they made us change how we thought about doing or eating things we'd always done or eaten. Yet we both found that, with each healthy change we made, it got easier and easier. Now our new ways of doing things are second nature.

So, pick a step that appeals to you, whether it's containing your plastic bags (chapter 36), finding an unscented laundry product (chapter 22), or choosing the organically-raised version of a food (chapter 66). Begin with that. Then try something more. Over the long term, a small consistent effort adds up to a very big difference, just as walking one step at a time can take you as far as you want to go, whether it's down the street or around the world!

If it appeals to you, find a friend who is also interested in making healthy changes and buddy up so you can encourage each other, share discoveries, and discuss the process with a sympathetic listener.

This book is designed to so you can read it straight through or skip around to chapters that catch your interest and work with them first. Whichever method you choose, take action! No matter how small, every positive step you take counts.

At the end of the book is a Resource Guide to help you source products or services mentioned in the text. This chapter and the next four will introduce you to concepts that are referred to throughout the book and provide you with a toolkit of ideas to keep in mind when making choices on your journey of health.

Let's begin this journey with your immune system.

The immune system is amazing! Until I started to learn about health, I had no idea it was so important. I used to think my immune system lounged around in my body waiting until I got sick to leap into action, like an internal superhero. Wrong!

The immune system does act to heal you when you're sick but it also works hard when you're *not* sick. Its regular job is to keep your body in a state of homeostasis, or balance, so you don't get sick in the first place. When you lose your homeostasis, you break down, your organs stop functioning properly, and eventually you die.

This doesn't happen overnight. Your body may spend years struggling to stay in balance before there is serious deterioration. The symptoms I described having in the first chapter are examples of the struggle to stay in balance. This struggle grows harder and more uncomfortable as the years go by.

But you don't have to settle for deterioration and discomfort. Unlike a machine, your body has the remarkable capacity to heal itself, especially when you take health-supporting action. That's why it is important to do everything possible to make life easy on your immune system. The ideas in this book have one simple goal: to *support the immune system* and help your body stay healthy.

Your immune system is like a watchdog. It guards your homeostasis day and night and checks out everything that comes your way, physical or emotional. No matter what substances you eat, drink, breathe or rub onto your skin, the watchdog wants to know if the molecules of these substances are friends or trouble-makers.

Friendly molecules or substances support your immune function and bring your body hydration, fiber, oxygen, and nutrients. Problem substances alert the watchdog to take protective action. Your immune system sees them as stresses or *toxins*. The more time your watchdog spends on alert, protecting you from toxins, the more you become overstressed and exhausted.

You can make life a lot easier for you and your immune system by reducing, eliminating, and avoiding toxins. Reducing exposure is important because your body usually deals with more than one toxin at the same time. Call these combined toxins your *total toxic load* and imagine it as a load of bricks you carry around all day. A heavy load makes it hard for you to keep your homeostasis and good health. On the other hand, when you start removing and avoiding toxic bricks, you lighten the burden on your immune system. The lighter your toxic burden, the better you feel.

But how do you recognize when there are too many bricks?

2. RECOGNIZING YOUR BODY'S MESSAGES.

Your body is smart. It knows the difference between toxins and healthy stuff. It knows exactly what causes trouble for it. The problem it has is how to get the message out to *you*. If you're like I was, you may not know what the message looks like. You may not even think there *is* a message.

There are a couple of ways to tune in to your body's messages. Services that test for your reactions are one option. (Reactions to substances will be called 'intolerance' or 'sensitivity'.) Another option is to pay attention.

But pay attention to what? Below is a list of possible messages from your body. Check off any you have on a regular basis. Remember, we're not talking here about the fatigue you feel after exercise or a stressful day, or about the occasional indigestion or irritability you experience. Think in terms of repeated or chronic messages. Especially pay attention to any signal or message you're so used to, you've come to think it's normal.

Message from your body:
☐ headache ☐ fatigue ☐ coughing ☐ shortness of breath ☐ frequent colds and flu ☐ joint pain ☐ skin problems ☐ can't concentrate ☐ memory problems ☐ bags or shadows under eyes ☐ food cravings ☐ addictive behaviors ☐ constipation ☐ diarrhea ☐ indigestion ☐ flatulence ☐ frequent urination ☐ menstrual problems ☐ yeast infections ☐ clumsiness ☐ muscle weakness ☐ irritability ☐ rage ☐ depression ☐ weepiness ☐ roller coaster emotions ☐ hyperactivity ☐ hypersensitivity ☐ behavior and/or learning problems ☐ other reactions I have:

Now look over the messages you have checked off and think about how often you feel this way. Is it once a day? More often? Once or several times a week? Once a month? Is it during one or more seasons? Spring and autumn, for example? Late summer, or part of the winter? Do you feel this way after a particular meal or after working with a certain type of product? Or when you're with a specific person? Do any of your blood relatives share your reactions? How long have you had these reactions and when did they begin? Since childhood? After a job change or house renovation? Think in terms of your emotional and mental reactions as well as the physical ones.

Once you start to pay attention to yourself, you'll notice little things that weren't apparent before. That irritation you feel after a trip to the dry cleaner, your indigestion and gas after meals, the inexplicable fatigue that overwhelms you in the autumn when the cold weather comes and the furnace goes on, your six-year-old's need to pee every time you've just driven away from the gas station, the headaches your husband has after the new carpet is installed—all of these are messages about toxic overload. Too many bricks!

We all have some illness or injury in the course of our lives. But many health problems can be prevented or corrected before they become serious. Prevention is *always* less costly than treating serious (acute) or chronic illness, whether you count the cost in dollars, physical pain, time spent being ill or undergoing treatment, psychological and emotional stress, or the freedom to do the things you want to do when you want to do them.

When you pay attention to your body's signals of toxic overload you gain the chance to take health-supporting action. And you will be able to measure the success of your action because the signals will fade or disappear. The checklist in this chapter, and the questions below it, can help you learn to recognize your body's messages and discover your own patterns of reaction. As you read through this book, you can refer back to the list to help you choose which health-supporting steps you will act on first.

3. BUT NOTHING BOTHERS ME! MASKING.

What if you have some messages from your body but you think that's just the way life goes? Maybe you feel okay most of the time and believe nothing bothers you. You could be right, especially if you have great genes, a fabulous environment, and terrific health habits, or other mitigating factors. Or you could be *masking*.

Masking is a coping mechanism for dealing with repeated exposures to toxins. It happens because your body will do *anything* to keep you in balance and maintain your homeostasis. To make sure you survive, your body will use up all its nutrients, enzymes, and water to neutralize and expel toxins so everything appears normal. This appearance of normality is called masking. When you're still healthy, you won't even be aware of this desperate use of your own resources.

Here's how it works. Imagine you just breathed in a chemical vapor. Your immune system sounds the alarm, registering the chemical as a toxin. You sneeze and cough, the smell of the chemical makes you recoil, and you feel dizzy, angry or develop a headache.

Now, imagine you have to spend time with that chemical every day, perhaps because you work with it. After a while you "get used to it" and stop having the initial signals of alarm. In reality, your body is no happier about the toxic exposure than it was the first time, but now it is masking your true reaction to get you through the day.

Masking is tremendously demanding. It is really a kind of life or death struggle. Will the toxins win or will your body be able to continue neutralizing them? The problem is, your body needs the nutrients and enzymes it uses up on masking for other processes, like building cells, healing injuries, keeping the nervous system in shape, and handling your daily physical and mental stresses. After years of masking, one day your body may be too worn out to continue with it any more. This is when people find out they have a life-threatening disease that developed "overnight" or, equally devastating, their brains don't function correctly any more.

You can find out if you're masking the effects of a substance by staying away from it for a few days. A re-exposure after that break will show your body's true reaction. (See chapters 67-69.) Professional testing services are another option. (More on this in chapter 67, *Testing for sensitivities.*)

We live in a culture that teaches us *not* to listen to our bodies, but to treat them like machines that can be fixed or replaced when they break down. We learn to ignore our symptoms or seek temporary relief that does nothing to address the underlying cause of trouble. Some younger bodies are able to remain healthy no matter what they are exposed to, because they are so efficient at masking. But with increased toxins in the environment, even the young are losing the struggle to neutralize toxins and are less and less healthy.

Even if nothing seems to bother you now, don't let masking fool you out of supporting your health.

4. TOXINS: THE DEAL AND THE REAL.

Is this toxin business really such a big deal? We all know of someone who lived to age 90 on a diet of cigars and whiskey. The comedian George Burns is a classic example. In every generation, there are a few people with a huge capacity for processing toxins that would flatten others.

Most of us do better to err on the side of caution. Clinical ecologists—physicians who specialize in environmental effects on health—point out that toxins in food, air, water, and products contribute to the current epidemics of asthma, allergies, and A.D.D. in the young as well as fibromyalgia, chronic fatigue, liver and kidney damage, and cancer in many age groups. So toxins *are* a big deal and avoiding them is the practical choice.

There are different groups of toxins. Some substances are toxic to *everyone* and have quick and obvious results that tend to be fatal: cyanide, arsenic, and nuclear radiation fall into this category.

Other toxins are less apparent and may only show their effects on you after they've been in your life for some time. Chemicals make up much of this group: pesticides in food, chemical ingredients in personal care and household products, air pollution, solvents, and weed killers are a few examples. Radiation and repressed emotions, though not substances, can have similar negative effects. In our stressful industrialized world, there are lots of toxins to choose from!

Then there are substances that are toxins for some people but not others. These include pollen, pet hair, various foods, mold, and dust. This group is sometimes called the classic allergens.

Common allergens can act as toxins for people with no known allergies. Medical doctors Stuart Berger and Doris Rapp report unrecognized toxic effects on many non-allergic people from the following allergens: chemical products, scented products, dairy, wheat, corn, sugar, caffeine, peanuts, yeast, oranges and orange juice, eggs, pork, shellfish, food additives, and food colors.

A curious fact about the foods on this list is that they typically contain high levels of pesticides, antibiotics, chemical residues, molds, hybridization, dyes or pollutants. Whether it is the foods themselves or these other components that provoke the body's negative reaction is still a question for researchers. Some people seem to be fine with foods from organic (chemical-free) sources even though they react to the conventionally-grown product. Coffee is a typical example.

Some toxins act as *neurotoxins,* which means they alter the way signals between body and brain travel and are interpreted, affecting emotions, thoughts, and behavior patterns. Neurotoxins may cause depression, rage, forgetfulness, lack of coordination, dyslexia, hyperactivity or confusion, to name only a few possibilities. Neurotoxins are probably more common than we realize, since they come with familiar foods or products.

At this point, you may be thinking that everything in your life has just been listed as a toxin. Don't worry! For every situation or product that harms your health, there's a safer, cleaner version, or a way to reduce your exposure. This book explains how.

5. GOOD STUFF IN; BAD STUFF OUT.

In chapter 1, we talked about the importance of supporting your immune system so it can keep you healthy. Avoiding toxins is one way you can provide this support, but avoidance tactics are not your only option. Actually, it's simple. To support your immune system, all you need to do is follow this equation: *good stuff in; bad stuff out.*

Good stuff is safe products, toxin-free water and air, safe furnishings and clothing, high quality nutrients, enzymes, restful sleep, relaxation, exercise, fun, and laughter. Bad stuff is harmful chemicals, toxic products, polluted air and water, foods that disagree with you, mold (mycotoxins), and negative stress or what Hans Selye, father of stress research, calls "distress".

Since you can't control the entire planet (much as some of us might like to), don't worry about it. The most important environment for you to control is your own home. When you make your house into a health-supporting oasis free from the toxins and pollutants in the outside world, you give your immune system a huge boost.

Home is where it really counts to do everything you can to support your immune system. That's because you probably spend a lot of time in your house. If not, chances are you at least sleep there, and sleep is the time when your body does much of its healing and repair work. If you are sleeping—or doing anything else—in a house full of toxins, your healing and repairing can end up on the sidelines while your body copes with your toxic surroundings. Illness, chronic health problems, and rapid aging are possible outcomes.

No one I know has a perfect equation of bringing only good stuff into their lives while getting all the bad stuff out. Perfection is not a useful measurement for most of us. What works better is to think in terms of loading up on the positive side. When you make your home into a pollution-free oasis and choose health-supporting personal care products, furnishings, and clothing, you create some room to play with what goes into your body (chocolate). Unless you are already ill. Adding good stuff into your life will create health improvements even *before* you take out the bad stuff. And doing both will give you the best possible results.

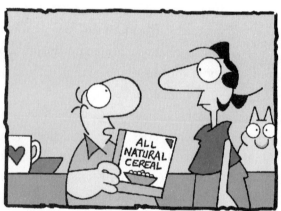

"The cavemen ate food that was 100% natural and their average life span was only 30 years."

A word here about our title, *How to Stay Healthy and still Eat Chocolate.* For "chocolate", you can substitute your own favorite food or drink. Whatever your favorite may be, we are not recommending that you indulge to excess or ingest foods or other substances you know are hard on you, even harmful! Instead, our idea is that when you clear your life of most toxins and you practice health-supporting actions, you can handle some chocolate or coffee or whatever. On the other hand, if you're surrounded by bad stuff and don't bring good stuff into your life, chocolate or any other treat may become the toxic brick that pushes your health over the edge. The lower your total toxic load, the less likely one brick is to topple you.

The following chapters will show you many ways to recognize and reduce bad stuff, choose good stuff, and create a healthy balance. First we'll look at personal care products, laundry and clothing choices, and home remedies, then at how to make your home into a toxin-free haven, and finally, at food, water, and other factors that contribute to your good health.

Note: See Resource Guide at end of book to locate products.

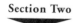

PERSONAL CARE

6. WHAT GOES ON YOUR SKIN GOES INTO YOUR BODY.

A good place to start choosing good stuff is with personal care products and cosmetics since they go right on your skin and stick there all day. When buying these products, I use this guideline: if I'm afraid to get it in my mouth, I don't want it on my skin. Fortunately, there are *lots* of products on the market that are user-friendly, as more and more companies move to organic and plant-based ingredients. We'll look at these products over the next few chapters.

Why am I so picky about what I put on my skin? Until a few years ago, I thought my skin was a barrier, a protective covering that kept everything outside out. Whatever touched my skin stayed right there and went no deeper. Or so I thought! I've since learned I'm not the only one to believe this common fallacy

The truth is, your skin both eliminates and absorbs. Skin absorbs so effectively that you can think of it this way: if you rub it on your skin, you're eating it. After World War II, when concentration camp survivors had trouble digesting food because of their years of starvation, they were able to receive nutrients by having liquid vitamins rubbed onto their skins. These days, patients wear drug patches to release medication into their bodies through the skin over the course of several hours. So the same thing can happen with anything you put on your skin.

It was also after World War II that the petrochemical industry took off. Since then, thousands of chemicals have been synthesized annually and are made into products we use, which releases them into the environment. According to William J. Rea, M.D., founder and director of the Environmental Health Center-Dallas, in the 30 years after 1965, four million chemical compounds were reported, with about 6,000 new ones being added every year!

Few chemicals are adequately tested for their long-term consequences to living beings. Synthetic chemicals are implicated in such diseases and dangerous physical changes as cancer, hormone disruption, and genetic mutation, which take years to develop or may only show their effects in children and following generations. While some chemicals are considered "non-toxic", that in itself is a questionable term.

Chemical products can act as neurotoxins, affecting the way you think, feel and behave. If you have headaches, feel depressed, lose your temper or forget things easily, you may be suffering the neurotoxic effects of chemical exposure. Research scientist Dr. J. Robert Hatherill associates heavy metals in pollutants with violent behavior and the growing problem of adolescent deliquency and homicide. Men are increasingly at risk of sterility through exposure to chemical toxins in products and the surrounding environment.

Children's products are no less suspect. They may be labeled "tearless" and so forth, but unless they are actually organic-source, unscented products, they are bound to contain chemicals. Toxic overload may explain the epidemic of learning, behavior, and breathing problems in today's children.

So, is there any hope for us in the face of all this terrifying information? Absolutely! Despite the many chemicals out there, what you choose to put on your skin and scalp can make a huge difference to your physical body, mind, and emotions.

When you switch to natural source, toxin-free personal care products, you enjoy a wonderful lifting of the toxic burden on your body and brain. Your immune system will no longer have to struggle to clear toxins from your body. Your liver and kidneys can have a break from working overtime to eliminate chemical residues. (Long-term exposure to pollutants may be just as damaging to the liver as heavy drinking.)

Chemicals have a tendency to store in fat cells but you don't have to let them stay there! You can sweat them out in a sauna. Udo Erasmus, Ph.D., author of *Fats that Heal, Fats that Kill*, says studies on soldiers exposed to Agent Orange showed they were able to expel even this horrible mutagenic poison from their cells with the sauna method. If you don't have access to a sauna, try a steam bath or any activity that makes you sweat. To further release toxins, eat foods that act to bind and expel chemicals, particularly green vegetables and sea vegetables like dulse or kelp. Erasmus also suggests EFA-rich oils help protect you from chemical toxins. (See chapter on *essential fatty acids*.)

Perhaps you would like to reduce your chemical exposure so you won't have toxins collecting in your body in the first place. One way to do this is to take a look at all your personal care products. Examine your toothpaste, soaps, shampoo, conditioner, hair spray, cosmetics, creams and lotions, hair removers, shaving cream, cologne and aftershave, bath products, body powders, nail products, and products containing fragrance. All these products come in contact with your skin. What ingredients are listed on their labels?

Health-supporting products will contain ingredients such as: water, herbs and other plants and their oils, aloe vera, tea tree oil, vegetable glycerine, vitamins, minerals, honey, beeswax, sea salt, and baking soda (sodium bicarbonate). If you see a petrochemical ingredient such as methyl/propyl paraben, the closer it is to the end of the list, the less of it is in the product. Choosing a mostly natural product with a tiny amount of chemical will be much better for your health than an all chemical product.

A partial list of chemical ingredients includes: fluoride, fragrance, artificial colors, ethanol, paraffin, plastics, polyethylene, acrylates, BHA, BHT, isopropyl alcohol, phenol, aerosol propellants, propylene glycol, parabens, vinyl, words with two-digit numbers after them, and anything with such a long name you can't even pronounce it let alone spell it! If you're not really sure what's in your personal care products, try asking in the store where you bought them. My personal experience is that the stores with healthier products tend to have more information for me about the ingredients in their merchandise.

If your personal care products are mostly made of chemicals, you may decide they are too dangerous to keep. In that case, grit your teeth, go through your house, collect all these products and give or throw them away. (Some can only be disposed of at your local toxic waste facility. See the chapter called *Discover your local toxic waste dump*.) Or use up what you already own and when each item is finished, replace it with a health-safe version.

When you put safe products on your skin, you protect yourself from wearing and absorbing dangerous chemicals that store up in your tissues and organs. Over the next few chapters, we'll look at health-supporting choices in various personal care products. For help locating products, check our Resource Guide at the end of the book.

7. DOES PERFUME DRIVE YOU WILD?

My husband used to go wild when I put on perfume. Wild with breathing problems.

Scented products are a problem for *everyone*, not just for people who *know* they're perfume-sensitive. There are a couple of reasons for this.

First, the scents in most products you buy contain chemicals, *hundreds* of them, including formaldehyde. Formaldehyde is used to preserve dead bodies. Yuck! Only plant-based products and botanical-source essential oils are free of chemical toxins.

The chemicals in perfumes often act as neurotoxins, meaning they affect your nervous system and the way signals pass between your brain and body. Look back at the reactions you checked off on the list in chapter 3. Have you experienced any of the following? Mood swings, depression, headaches and dizziness, fuzzy headedness, irritability, sudden angry outbursts, and lack of coordination are all neurotoxic symptoms of perfume sensitivity. Multiple sclerosis is a disorder of the central nervous system. Physical perfume reactions you might experience are food cravings, skin or bowel problems, menstrual trouble or fatigue. And even if the perfume you wear doesn't seem to irritate *you*, others, including your children, could react to it with behavior and health problems.

A second reason perfume may be a problem comes from my former teacher, Sherry. Here's her theory:

As humans moved through the millenia, trying to upgrade themselves from the primeval ooze, the only available perfume arrived during blossom season when flowers scented the air. Blossom season is short. So for thousands of years, these few months would be the extent of most people's perfume exposure.

Now, through the inventiveness of the chemical industry, you can surround yourself with a cloud of perfume 24 hours a day, seven days a week, 365 days a year. Total full-time exposure equals *overexposure*. This artificial extension of the natural season creates problems for many people, who remain perfume sensitive even around totally natural plant-source scents, perhaps because their bodies have learned to associate scent with trouble and cannot distinguish between the natural and the artificial.

Why does this happen? Imagine being with your spouse *all* the time, no breaks, no time to yourself—ever. How long before the trouble begins? It's the same with perfume, or anything to which you receive too much exposure.

So, if you've been driving yourself wild with perfume, take a break. Give your body a chance to breathe and learn how it feels to be clean without being scented. Then use perfume judiciously. Go about your regular day unscented. Use a natural-source essential oil product for special occasions, or apply a little vanilla extract behind your ears. Put your old chemical perfumes in a box and store them in the garage. Try a little on a special occasion, if you wish, but see how you feel—if you get a headache or intestinal gas or drink considerably more than you normally would, you're probably reacting to your perfume.

The truth is, it's not the perfume you wear that drives the opposite sex wild, it's the hormones and chemicals produced by your own body! Being your natural self is really the sexiest—and healthiest—thing you can do.

8. SOAP.

Hand and body soaps can be full of harsh chemicals including formaldehyde, ammonia, preservatives, and fragrance that dry out the skin and add to the body's toxic load. Deodorant soaps in particular are questionable, and have not been proven any more effective at cleaning the body or eliminating odors than plain soap. Children, with their developing immune systems, should *never* use them. Anti-bacterial or bactericidal soaps may contain benzene, a carcinogen, and are currently being tested for possible dioxin contamination.

The chemicals in soap may be absorbed directly into the skin and from there throughout the body, where they lodge in the organs. Use of any soap that causes a burning or unpleasant sensation to the genital area or other delicate skin should be discontinued immediately, even if it is a natural soap.

Products—especially soaps and deodorants—available in regular grocery and drug stores are not always unscented even when this word appears on the package. They may lack the heavy fragrance added to the usual version of the product, yet have a powerful chemical odor. When I trustingly bought the "unscented" version of a well-known soap and almost choked from the smell, I was able to return it for a refund.

Look for unfragranced bar or liquid soap that is glycerin or vegetable-based. You can buy this kind of soap at the natural foods store and at some grocery and drug stores. Nature Clean, available at all types of stores, makes both bar and liquid hand and body soap that is truly unscented. Avalon Organics makes a wonderful plant-scented liquid soap. When buying soaps, always read the label or ask the store about the ingredients (if there is no packaging). Beware of soaps made by companies who do not freely disclose their product ingredients.

Glycerin and olive oil soaps tend to have more lubricating qualities than other soaps. Any soap made of pure vegetable materials without added scent will be gentle on skin, so it's safe to use on your face, and easy on your health.

If you have been washing your face with soap, no matter how elegant, then using moisturizer to correct dryness, try washing with only water. Use a washcloth, to stimulate your skin's circulation and remove dead surface cells.

Soap is drying to the skin, and any soap or cleanser may be too much for the delicate skin of the face. Unless you have extremely oily skin, you may not require soap to clean your face, particularly after your teen years.

9. HOW TO SAFELY CLEAN GASOLINE OR OTHER STRONG CHEMICALS OFF YOUR SKIN.

Say the worst happens. You're at the gas station and you accidentally spill some gas on your hands. You try wiping it off with paper towel, but the smell remains. You run into the washroom and wash your hands with soap, but you can still smell the gas.

At this point, you wonder what kind of powerful cleaner or solvent you can buy to solve the problem. Then you remember that everything you put on your skin is absorbed into your body and migrates to your organs. Maybe the available cleaners and solvents will be deadlier than what you spilled on your hands in the first place!

What to do?

All you really need is baking soda. Carry a small bottle of it in your car for gas station emergencies. If you have any natural soap available, lather up, then sprinkle a good dose of baking soda onto your hands and rub it into the affected area. You can let this mixture sit for a couple of minutes. If you have no soap, just use baking soda. Baking soda is a natural deodorizer and will absorb smells while it cleans.

If the smell is very strong, you may need to rub the area with a slice of lemon or squeeze fresh lemon juice over it as a sort of finishing rinse, after you have washed off the baking soda. The gas and the smell will be gone. Even without the lemon, baking soda usually removes the smell of gas from skin.

If you get an oil-based product like asphalt driveway sealer on your skin, wash it off with a grease-cutting dish soap. I easily cleaned my cat's feet with the Soap Factory's biodegradable dish liquid after she walked across our freshly-sealed driveway. Cats are *very* chemically-sensitive—much more so than humans—and quickly absorb toxins through the pads of their paws, so *never* use solvents or harsh cleansers on them. Ecover dish soap is another excellent choice.

These cleaning solutions can be applied if you spill paint or grease on yourself. They won't harm your skin or your long-term health! If you're using a chemical product and you're concerned about getting it on your skin, cover up with long sleeves and trousers and wear gloves.

10. HAIR CARE.

As with soap, chemicals in shampoos and conditioners are absorbed directly into the skin. Shampoo may contain detergent, plastics, sulphur compounds, the same chemicals listed for soap, and a few other toxic goodies. One of the most common toxins in both shampoo and soap is the coloring agent! These colors are made from coal tar and have mostly all proven to be carcinogenic. Shampoo may also contain sodium laurel sulphate. Dandruff shampoos are particularly toxic.

Look for unfragranced, uncolored (or naturally-colored) shampoos, and conditioners. Nature Clean, Simply Clear from The Soap Factory, and Infinity are three unscented, bio-friendly brands. You can also substitute pure liquid soap for shampoo, although it may not feel quite the same on your hair.

Ferlow Brothers of British Columbia makes top quality unscented shampoos that use only herbal, non-chemical ingredients. They require no conditioner. Clinique makes a full line of unscented, color-free hair care products including shampoo, conditioner, gel, and hairspray, available at department stores. Aveda products are heavily plant-based, and are low enough in petrochemical derivatives that your exposure is minimal. Ask specifically for their fragrance- and color-free line called "All-Sensitive".

Never assume a product is fragrance-free unless it *specifically* says so. Products that say "natural" on the label are not necessarily fragrance-free. Read the ingredient list to make sure, even in the natural foods store. The word "fragrance" is usually mentioned somewhere near the end of the list and is easy to overlook. If the only word listed on the label is "fragrance" or "scent", *always* assume this indicates a chemical source and do not buy the product.

If you *do* decide to go with a fragranced product, make sure the scent is from a plant (botanical) source rather than a petrochemical one. Plant-source scents are listed as such and the particular plants or botanicals will be named (e.g. lavender, rosemary, lemon, etc.) Avalon Organics, Nature's Blends, and Prairie Naturals make excellent plant-scented products. The first two include certified organic ingredients.

For dandruff, try baking soda. Chronic dandruff is often related to some type of food or chemical sensitivity, which must be addressed before the scalp condition will clear. If you have high-level nutrition and enough essential fatty acids in your diet, dandruff should not be a problem (see chapter 16, *Real skin food*, and chapters 74 to 76 on Fats and Oils.)

When choosing a hairspray, go for the non-aerosol version in the pump bottle, not a spray can. Aerosol propellants in spray cans are extremely damaging to your health and to the environment. Marcelle and Clinique are good choices.

When I go to a salon to have my hair cut, I take along my own natural and unscented shampoo, conditioner, and hair spray for them to use on me. I have never had a problem with a salon when I do this, especially when I explain that I react badly to perfumed products. What typically happens is the staff gathers around to examine the products and to learn what is special about them.

Even taking this precaution, you may react badly to the chemicals in the air at a salon. When scheduling appointments, ask if there will be anyone having a perm or manicure at the same time, so you can avoid being around those highly toxic chemicals. You may decide to look for a salon specializing in organic and nontoxic hair care, perhaps one that carries Aveda or another botanical product line, or one that has installed excellent air filtration so the toxic chemicals do not circulate in the salon air.

Hair dyes should NEVER be used on children. Dyes aren't good for adults either! Of all hair products, they are the most dangerous and the least controlled. They contain mutagens and suspected carcinogens, as well as chemicals which have not been tested for safety. Among the toxic brew of ammonia, fragrance, detergents, colors, ethanol, glycols, and sulfur compounds, is *lead*, which can cause permanent neurological damage, behavior alterations, and brain damage. Lead is so toxic, it harms literally *every* system in the body.

Hair coloring is a risky business, so if you choose to do it, protect yourself by looking for the safest possible products, or using only methods where the dye does not touch your scalp. Women who use chemical dyes may be at increased risk for breast and other cancers. If you are going prematurely grey (sooner than other members of your blood family), you may be suffering from too much stress, or lack nutrients, essential fatty acids, and fresh leafy greens in your diet.

Women who are pregnant or considering pregnancy should avoid hair dyes. That means *young women who have not yet had their children should stay as far away from hair dye as possible.* Don't take chances with your family's genetic heritage! At least wait until after your children are born before you start dying your hair.

The most dangerous processes tend to be the most extreme. For example, if you have dark hair and decide to go blond or red, this involves bleaching your hair before the lighter color is applied. Bleach on your head makes for neurotoxic, possible carcinogenic, and other health damaging effects.

When you go to a salon, ask about the ingredients in the product(s) being used on your head. For home hair coloring, check products available in natural foods stores, the Body Shop, or try traditional herbal methods.

11. DEODORANT.

In his *Extraordinary Origins of Everyday Things*, Charles Panati explains that chemical deodorants don't work for very long, despite their claims! The reason for this has to do with sweat glands and how they're arranged on your body.

There are two types of sweat gland: eccrine and apocrine. The eccrine are spread all over the body. They help you to cool off in hot sun or while exercising. The apocrine glands are located mostly in the armpit. Some eccrine glands are in the armpit too, but it's the apocrine that are largely responsible for underarm odor.

Now comes the bizarre part. Apparently, chemical sweat gland blockers in deodorants block *only* the eccrine glands! I guess that leaves perfume or luck to cover up the smell from the apocrines! Or maybe deodorants work through the power of suggestion, like placebos. Who knows! This gland business explains why some people search endlessly for a deodorant that "works", turning to stronger and stronger brands, without success.

Stress, nervousness, and our speeded-up pace of life make some body odor normal for everyone. But continual severe body odor can be a sign of internal trouble caused by disease, poor nutrition, allergies or sensitivities to foods and chemicals, or alcoholism. When your body is trying to eliminate serious toxins, major body odor can result. If you go on a cleanse or suddenly improve your diet and lifestyle, you may experience some unusual temporary body odor as your system cleans itself out.

Apart from aluminum or zinc for dryness, chemical deodorants contain toxic ingredients including formaldehyde, fragrance, colors, ammonia, and ethanol. If they are sprays (unless they come in pump format), they contain aerosol propellants. This is hardly a safe product to be applying to the delicate skin of the underarm, particularly after shaving.

Safer alternatives include the deodorant stone, baking soda, and natural roll-on or stick deodorants. Avalon Organics makes a plant-scented roll-on. Earthwise brand or other deodorant sticks containing baking soda or sodium bicarbonate are effective. Deodorant stones are an actual mineral stone. The concept is simple and elegant, however, as with all deodorants, they don't work for everyone. The only way to find out is to try one. If you feel that natural deodorants are not strong enough for you, try hypo-allergenic deodorants available in pharmacies and department stores. These will be scent-free.

A piece of anecdotal evidence about deodorant: A woman we know decided to protect her health by changing to a natural deodorant instead of the chemical version she had been using. After she threw away the chemical product, she noticed red, swollen lumps in both underarms that lasted for several weeks. Although she was in perfectly good health, these strange lumps concerned her, so she consulted her doctor. The doc's verdict? Ingrown hairs!

Our friend wasn't so sure. Could she really have ingrown hairs in *both* underarms, making two lumps of the *same* size, in *exactly* the same place? She did a little research on her own and concluded the lumps were probably lymph glands. She figured they had swollen because they were detoxing her old deodorant, something that could finally occur because she'd stopped the daily chemical onslaught. After a while, the lumps simply went away with no further recurrence.

12. REAL SKIN FOOD.

Real skin food does not come in a cosmetic pot. The older men and women I know who have the best skin are life-long exercisers, often practitioners of yoga. Any aerobic exercise that stimulates oxygenation and circulation and reduces stress benefits skin.

What makes skin go bad? Stress, pollution, sugar, alcohol, flour products, caffeine, heated and processed fats, and smoking. Smoking increases wrinkles especially around the mouth and may encourage enlarged pores.

High intake of sweets is another factor in the destruction of skin quality. Israeli lab tests show that fructose intake over time increases collagen loss, leading to collagen breakdown in older people. Collagen is a protein that helps to keep skin supple by supporting the production of connective tissue. So the more sweets you eat, the more wrinkled your skin will be.

The sun is often blamed for skin destruction, yet some sunlight in moderation is vital to skin quality. Puffy eyes and dark circles under the eyes are very often a sign of food or other allergy. And as we all know, lack of sleep and relaxation is a killer for the skin.

What benefits skin? Exercise and meditation can work wonders, at any stage in life. Real skin food includes sufficient protein, lots of vitamin-rich vegetables and fruit, filtered water, and top-quality oils that supply the correct ratio of essential fatty acids. One product that provides this ratio is Udo's Ultimate Oil Blend, marketed by Flora, Inc. Another good source is any properly processed hempseed oil, such as Mum's certified organic oil from Biohemp Ltd. (see chapters on fats for more information.)

Udo Erasmus, author of *Fats that Heal, Fats that Kill*, points out that essential fatty acids (EFAs) are vital to internal processes and brain function. In fact, EFAs are so important, the body and brain will utilize any available for survival. You can easily survive with dry skin but you wouldn't last long without a heart rate, digestion or other life-supporting processes, so skin comes last on the list in receiving essential fatty acids. According to Udo, you will know when you get your diet and fat intake right because you will have soft, velvety skin, even in winter. This means that all your other organs are receiving the nutrients they need, so there are enough left over for the skin.

Another factor that determines women's skin quality is, of course, hormones. Young women have young skin in part because of their higher estrogen levels. Soy products, often recommended as a natural source of estrogens for menopausal women, may be useful as a skin nutrient (but eat them, don't put them on your face).

My personal favorite skin enhancer is laughter. Scientist Susan Everson of the Public Health Institute in Berkeley, California, says despair increases narrowing of the arteries, cardiovascular problems, and levels of stress hormones. And Shakespeare calls grief "beauty's canker." Well, if that's so, the opposite must be true—fun and laughter must improve your heart function, circulation, and relieve stress. My theory is the more you laugh, the better your skin will be. Call me crazy, but at least you'll have fun finding out!

13. POWDERS, CREAMS, AND MOISTURIZERS.

Powders:
Body powders can have a couple of health hazards: synthetic scent with its chemical mystery ingredients, and talc, which can be contaminated with asbestos. Asbestos is a known carcinogen.

A safe and inexpensive alternative is cornstarch. If you're sensitive to corn, try arrowroot powder or sifted organic oat flour. For a deodorizing effect, add a little baking soda. Baking soda is mildly abrasive, so don't add too much, especially if the powder is for a baby or child. A spoonful of baking soda to half a cup of flour or cornstarch should do it. Test it on yourself first.

Natural foods stores sell powders made from non-toxic ingredients, many of which use cornstarch or arrowroot as a base. Check the label to be sure the product you purchase is talc-free. Healthy Home Services offers a talc-free baby powder. The Body Shop carries an asbestos-free talc powder.

Creams and Moisturizers:

Clinique, Marcelle, and Almay make high-quality unscented facial moisturizers, and hand and body lotions. Aveda's All-Sensitive line offers an unscented moisturizer and a body oil that are primarily plant-based.

Muskoka Naturals offers a line of completely natural, synthetic-free skin care. Many natural foods stores now have cosmetic sections devoted to quality, plant-source products such as Ecco Bella and Avalon Organics. Some products have a mild scent because of the botanicals used in them, however, this is not the same as added synthetic fragrance. For example, Sonoma Soap Company makes a Pure Honey Hand Creme and a Body Lotion, both of which smell deliciously of the honey used in the formula but have no added fragrance.

Drug and department stores have a good selection of unscented hand and body lotions, both in the hypoallergenic cosmetic section and on the regular shelves. If your primary concern is to stop burdening your immune system with toxic scents, this is a good place to start. All the major lotion manufacturers—Lubriderm, Keri-lotion, etc.—have good unscented versions. However, if you are concerned about ingredients derived from a petrochemical source, you may want to move directly to using natural-source creams and lotions. Petrochemical derivatives include E.D.T.A. (or edetate) disodium, fragrance, alcohols, glyceryl, mineral oil, paraffin, and saccharin. Mineral oil, a common ingredient in body lotions and creams, interferes with your ability to absorb vitamins and is a suspected carcinogen, according to Debra Lynn Dadd.

Most products that are marketed as hypoallergenic can be returned if you have a negative reaction to them. Make sure they're marked "hypoallergenic" and not simply "unscented" or "fragrance-free". Ask, when making your purchase, if you're concerned about the return policy.

For extremely chapped hands, look for a hand cream that contains lanolin and beeswax, or apply straight olive oil to your hands. If necessary, soak your hands in slightly warm (room temperature) oil for a few minutes before blotting off with a dry washcloth. Or squeeze vitamin E from a capsule directly onto your hands as a restorative.

You can use food oils as body lotion or moisturizer. Pure almond, olive, avocado, macadamia or coconut oils are pleasant on the skin without having a strong smell. If you're sensitive or allergic to the food the oil comes from, don't use it.

The two best moisturizers of all are the ones that work from the inside: water—the water you drink—and essential fatty acids. As fats-and-oils authority Udo Erasmus says, when you eat the correct EFAs, your skin will always be soft and supple *without* moisturizers or creams!

14. COSMETICS. DO YOU REALLY HAVE TO SUFFER TO BE BEAUTIFUL?

Cosmetics go back thousands of years in human history and have always been safe or hazardous, depending on their ingredients. For over two thousand years, women and men used a lead-based powder to give themselves a fashionably pale complexion. The red for rouge and lip paint came from a mercury sulfide called cinnabar. Belladonna was used for eye drops. With such outright poisons applied straight to the body, it's a wonder the human race survived at all! These toxic beauty products must have resulted in many cases of brain damage, psychosis, neurological and physical disability, blindness, birth defects, miscarriage, and early death.

Today, lead and mercury are no longer a major ingredient in cosmetics, although they have not completely disappeared. We now lean heavily on the petrochemical industry for cosmetic and personal care products. Some of these petro-derivatives may be carcinogenic; some are implicated in the development of asthma as well as behavior and learning disorders. Many chemicals have not been adequately tested for their long-term effects on human health.

Cosmetic and personal care products, as well as all other products made with synthetic chemicals, are most frightening for their mutagenic potential. Mutagens may cause birth defects, fetal abnormalities, and cell changes that carry over into the next generation. The products a woman uses during her pregnancy affect her fetus, as do all the toxic chemicals that have stored in her tissues up until the time she became pregnant. So even if your children don't show a reaction to a product you used before they were born, *their* children can receive the ill effects. Unless you clear toxins out of your body, first. Dangerous ingredients include aerosol propellants, BHA and BHT, fluoride, formaldehyde, lead, polyvinyl chloride, and trichloroethylene. To protect your genetic future, you can sweat these chemicals out in a sauna or steam bath, detoxify with essential fatty acids, and eat lots of green vegetables and sea vegetables (seaweed) to help flush toxins out of your system. (More on this in later chapters.)

To keep from storing dangerous chemicals in your body in the first place, look for products that are low in petrochemical derivatives such as plastics, mineral oil, BHA and BHT, fragrance, synthetic colors and flavors, ammonia, paraffin, and saccharin. You may prefer to use products made from all, or almost all natural ingredients from plants. If you have allergies or sensitivities to a food, you'll also need to watch out for cosmetic ingredients from that food. Corn derivatives, wheat, dairy, sugar, peanut oil, and almond oil are possibilities.

Drug and department stores carry hypoallergenic lines such as Marcelle, Almay, and Clinique. You may want to check ingredient lists of individual products in these cosmetic lines to determine the amount of petro-derivatives. Bodies vary, therefore some products labelled 'hypoallergenic' may not work well for you, however, these products do tend to be unscented, which relieves a good portion of your total toxic load. You can usually return products marketed as hypoallergenic to the store if you find out you have a reaction to them.

Natural foods stores feature a vast array of cosmetics and personal care products, and more and more small manufacturers are springing up to bring you the latest in healthy make-ups. Ecco Bella makes a full range of plant-based cosmetics, sold in natural foods stores.

Here are some questions to ask when you are buying from an unfamiliar cosmetic line or considering a beauty treatment at a salon: what is the source of the ingredients—all natural plant sources or some petrochemical? Are the products fragranced and, if so, are they plant-derived scents? If essential oils are used, are any derived from chemical sources? Any reliable manufacturer will know the answers to these questions. You might also want to know the return policy for the cosmetics. If you have a means for testing the compatibility of the products for your body, ask if the seller will provide you with a small sample of the products you are interested in purchasing. (See the chapter on *Testing* for more information.)

15. REALITY CHECK: BUT I LOVE MY PERSONAL CARE PRODUCTS!

Before we go any farther with the personal care section, let's admit right here that you might feel resistance to some of this information. I did when I first heard it! I wanted better health and I wanted it to last. But the idea of clearing my house of all sorts of products I was used to and even *loved* was a bit much. In particular, I loved my perfume and my hair products. I just couldn't bring myself to get rid of them. Could my shampoo really be all that dangerous?

Since I was still in the process of clearing toxins out of me and my house, I had yet to experience the many positive changes to come. All I knew was that someone was trying to take away products I loved, while telling me I'd be better off without them. The fact that that someone was me didn't help matters a whole lot.

So I compromised. Instead of throwing *everything* away, I found a box and packed up all the stuff I loved that didn't love me back. I stored it in the garage, telling myself I'd leave it there for at least one month. Then I got started with all new unscented products, free of toxic chemicals. I could hardly wait for the day when I'd feel great again and could retrieve all my favorites.

But the strangest thing happened! A month passed, and then another month. I was feeling better and better all the time. I forgot about my nice products in the garage. When I finally *did* remember, I went out and opened the box. The odor almost knocked me over! I couldn't believe how *strong* everything smelled. I didn't want any of *that* on my skin or hair. It was obvious I'd be lost in a chemical fog the minute I used those products, followed by a renewal of my old symptoms—the sniffling, indigestion, roller coaster emotions, and so forth.

So, I gave all my old products away. And you know what? I've *never* missed them, not even once. When I think about what was in those products, I sometimes wonder how I survived them!

If you're like me, don't force yourself to throw everything away at once. Do clear your house of products mentioned in this book and put them in boxes for storage in your garage or somewhere where they can't affect your indoor air. This will lift a huge load from your immune system.

Then wait. Wait a good three months while you try out non-toxic and unscented products. See how you feel. Keep a journal if you wish and write down everything—physical changes, emotional and mental states. Do you still have frequent food cravings? What about PMS? Has that little morning cough gone away? Are you able to walk faster and not run out of breath the way you used to? Are you less irritable, depressed, confused? Have your headaches or skin problems cleared up? Take note.

After you have given the non-toxic and unscented products a fair trial, check out your old products again and observe what happens. You may never look back.

16. SUNSCREEN.

What about outdoor skin products? Sunscreen and suntan lotions were developed in the 1940's when American soldiers in the Pacific needed protection from tropical sun. They got it from red petrolatum, a petrochemical byproduct whose color blocked ultraviolet rays. Chemists evolved this into the white sunscreen we know today.

Using sunscreen means making choices about time and place. If you spend hours in the sun, you need protection from burning rays. But always covering up your skin with screening lotions prevents the sun exposure you need to make vitamin D and stimulate your immune system. You need *some* sun for good health, and not an overdose.

Prior to the 20th century, sun-darkened skin was unfashionable so people covered up with clothing, hats, parasols, and shade. Those prudent habits could be part of your sun strategy. Instead of coating yourself with petrochemical byproducts, monitor the amount of time you spend in direct sunlight, then move into the shade, or put on a hat, loose, long-sleeved top and lightweight pants, or a long cotton robe. Parasols and sun-umbrellas are useful too.

But *you must have a few minutes of unscreened exposure to the sun every day*. Without it, you may end up with osteoporosis, depression, reduced immune function, and Seasonal Affective Disorder (S.A.D.). It helps considerably if you get this unscreened sun exposure *without* wearing glasses or sunglasses. In some countries, women are required to wear the full veil with a fabric screen over the eyes. This prevents any direct sunlight from reaching their skin and eyes, making osteoporosis and osteomalacia (softening of the bones) very common.

When planning your sun time, take geography and skin type into account. People with more pigment in their skins may be able to spend more time in the sun safely than fair-skinned types. My friends of Mediterranean descent stay in the sun for hours and never burn. Whether this is fact or fallacy can be judged according to your health history—do you burn easily? Is there a history of skin cancer in your blood family? Did your ancestors come from sunny lands where they may have acclimatized to sun exposure or from cooler climates where rain and cloud often blocked the sun?

When it's bathing suit weather, give your skin time to get used to the sun's rays with short periods of exposure daily, especially if you've just spent the whole winter indoors or mostly covered up. Slowly build up the amount of time you spend in the direct sun, until you are able to be out without burning.

If you decide you need sunscreen, it is available at natural foods stores, or you can try an unscented version from the drugstore, such as Ombrelle. We've heard that plain sesame oil can prevent about 30% of harmful rays from reaching skin. Another alternative is to stay mostly indoors during the time of day when the sun's rays are at their peak—usually between about 10 a.m. and 2 p.m. This is especially important for children, who are more likely to spend hours in the sun than their parents. Have them go out when the rays are less intense, especially at the hottest time of year.

Another important factor in avoiding sunburn is to keep your nutrition at an optimal level. High-level nutrients protect and heal the skin. There's a theory that people who eat a lot of sugar and cooked fats burn more easily than those who eat lots of fresh, whole foods, raw fruits and vegetables, and the correct ratio of essential fatty acids. Could this be the reason those American servicemen needed sunscreen in the first place?

17. INSECT REPELLENT.

Insect repellents are pesticides and pesticides are toxic! Since we are already suffering major health problems from long-term pesticide build-up in our water and food supplies, it seems crazy to add to the danger by putting chemical insect repellent directly on our skins.

So what do you do if you happen to like outdoor activities and there are biting insects? There are several options. You can buy natural insect repellent made from mixtures of various oils such as citronella, tea tree, rosemary, and lemongrass. Try repellents by Thursday Plantation of Australia, Burt's Bees or Beebalm and Basil. The last two are safe to use on children and pets (remember that pets will lick whatever you put on them.) Burt's also makes Porch Incense whose smoke keeps insects away and Poison Ivy soap for hikers and gardeners who accidentally meet these unfriendly plants.

Citronella is a naturally-occuring scent bugs hate. In fact, there is a geranium you can buy called "mosquito geranium" which smells of citronella and is recommended for decks and patios, to keep insects away. If you like to experiment, you can make your own combination insect repellent and sunscreen by mixing pure sesame oil with tea tree oil and citronella oil. Buy citronella oil where essential oils are sold, or make your own by crushing leaves of mosquito geranium and soaking in sesame or olive oil.

Other oils that repel insects are lavender, geranium, and rosemary. All scented oils should be kept away from eyes and should be tested on a small patch of skin first, to see whether they are tolerated or will produce a rash. When buying essential oils, tell the clerk they are for use on skin and ask how much they should be diluted—you can mix them with sesame or olive oil, or your favorite unscented hand or body lotion.

A hiking friend found bug nets we could wear over our heads. These nets are very inexpensive, fit over hats, and are elasticized at the neck to keep insects out. They're not glamorous, but they work! I suspect, in centuries past, ladies' veils must have served the same purpose. In terms of remaining free of toxins, this is probably the best solution although it means covering arms and legs with clothing. Head-covering bug nets are available in hardware and sporting goods stores carrying small-boat fishing gear.

I've heard bugs are attracted to sweets and will hone in on people who have eaten a lot of sugar or sweet fruit, although this may be an urban myth. Anyone who has been in cottage country knows that mosquitoes have no prejudices when it comes to humans. However, like vampires, bugs dislike garlic so if you don't mind smelling garlicky, you can eat it or rub it on your skin. I've also heard that mosquitoes are attracted by our exhalations of carbon dioxide, so perhaps the smell of garlic breath confuses them. Garlic is a safe insect repellent to put on dogs. Never apply chemical insect repellents to dogs or cats as they lick their fur and will ingest the toxins directly.

Indoors, you can try mosquito geraniums in pots, or hang mosquito netting over your bed.

18. TOOTHPASTE AND FLUORIDE.

We've talked about skin. What about the stuff that goes right into your mouth, like fluoridated toothpaste? Fluoride is a chemical with a curious relationship to the body. *Calcium fluoride* occurs in nature and is important to bones and teeth in *very* tiny amounts, while *sodium fluoride*, which may be toxic, is the version used to fluoridate water. Charles Panati writes that as early as 1802, Neapolitan dentists noticed the cavity-preventing effects of naturally occuring fluoride in the local water. The cavity-free teeth reacted to the fluoride with yellowish brown spots which were unattractive but not a sign of decay.

In North America, sodium fluoride trials on drinking water for cavity prevention began in the early twentieth century, leading to fluoridation of oral hygiene products and municipal water. While this worked to help reduce cavities, other fluoride-related health problems occurred. Fluoride still causes spotty discoloration of teeth, as well as gum diseases and mouth ulcers—not a tremendously good record for a chemical that is supposed to encourage oral hygiene!

However, fluoride's effects range into far more dangerous categories. The chemical has been linked to several thousand deaths from cancer every year, as well as digestive problems including constipation and diarrhea, arthritis and asthma, skin and sinus problems, and vision disorders. Too much fluoride can bring about degeneration of heart, central nervous system, reproductive organs, liver, kidneys and adrenals, and suppress growth.

Fluoride and chlorine compete with iodine to fit into receptor sites in the thyroid gland, blocking thyroid function. The thyroid is usually 50% iodine. This vital gland regulates temperature in your body, affecting metabolism, body weight, and energy level. If all this isn't enough, fluoride is capable of causing genetic damage and weakens the immune system. There is some evidence to suggest that high levels of fluoridation in drinking water are related to an increase in Down's Syndrome. There must be better ways of fighting cavities!

According to Dr. Flora Parsa Stay in *The Complete Book of Dental Remedies*, fluoridated toothpaste is not the answer to preventing cavities. Brushing, flossing, and eating high nutrient foods is the way to do it. Outside of North America, most countries have banned the use of fluoride. Have your dentist clean your teeth with a non-fluoridated product.

Commercial toothpaste contains ingredients including sodium fluoride and formaldehyde that can be both mutagenic and carcinogenic. Other dangerous ingredients include ammonia—a respiratory tract and mucous membrane irritant, ethanol—which depresses the central nervous system, and mineral oil—a suspected carcinogen which prevents normal uptake of vitamins in the body.

There is even "antibacterial" toothpaste now, containing a biocide with the same damaging potential as any other pesticide!

Most natural foods stores carry a selection of fluoride-free, natural-source toothpastes such as Weleda, Nature's Gate, and Tom's of Maine. Tom's also sells a fluoridated version so read the label carefully.

Some natural toothpastes contain Australian tea-tree oil, which is antiseptic and antifungal. Peelu brand toothpaste is made from a tropical tree. The one caution with these tree-based products is for people who are sensitive to turpins, resins or tree pollen. If you know you have tree-related sensitivities or allergies, be careful about using tea-tree oil and Peelu products on a daily basis. Instead, try varying them with other products.

Sodium laurel sulphate is an ingredient in some toothpastes. There is controversy over whether or not natural-source sodium laurel sulphate is a carcinogen similar to synthetic sodium laurel sulphate. You have to make your own choice, but I am less worried about s.l.s. from coconuts than from chemicals.

Will natural toothpastes clean your teeth properly and keep them white, particularly when brighteners such as ammonia or titanium dioxide are not in the recipe? Actually it's thorough brushing and flossing of teeth that keeps them clean, not the toothpaste you use. According to Dr. Stay, harsh chemicals can make teeth sensitive.

And what about cavities? Will you get cavities if you don't use fluoride? The real cause of cavities is a diet high in refined carbohydrates and low in nutrients, along with poor dental hygiene. People who receive a good balance of vitamins and minerals and do not consume refined sugars and flours and processed foods tend to have cavity-free teeth. All forms of sugar promote the growth of bacteria in the mouth. (For more on how sweets affect tooth and bone formation, see chapters on Sugar.) Besides, if you live in an urban area, there's already enough fluoride in the water system that you'll never miss it on your toothbrush.

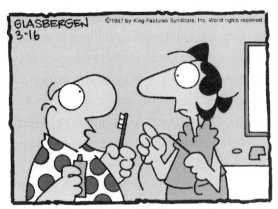

"My doctor told me to eat 5
fruits and vegetables every day.
Today I had 2 peas and 3 raisins."

19. MERCURY AMALGAM FILLINGS AND METAL IN YOUR MOUTH.

Do you have silver fillings? Well, guess what—they're not actually silver, they're an amalgam of mercury and several other metals. Mercury is a poison. Many dentists no longer use it, although, in North America, mercury is still not officially recognized by dental associations as a toxin!

Dr. Hal Huggins, author of *It's All In Your Head, The Link Between Mercury Amalgams and Illness*, says mercury in the body can stress the immune system so severely, it can cause serious disease states. He lists problems related to excess mercury ranging from irritation and indigestion, neurological and psychological disorders, to full-blown disease conditions. In order to help clear mercury from the body, he believes it is vital to eat sufficient protein, lipids (fats and oils), and in many cases to remove mercury fillings.

Although changing fillings is not always necessary or desirable, in *Prescription for Nutritional Healing*, Balch and Balch point out that chronic health problems are often resolved through removal of mercury amalgams.

Mercury accumulation can interfere significantly with your immune system. If you've had a long term condition—physical or emotional—that won't go away no matter what you do, you may want to reconsider your fillings.

If you decide to have your mercury amalgam fillings changed to composite or "white" fillings, ask some questions. When mercury fillings are removed, are patients and staff protected from mercury vapor with oxygen and/or masks? Is a dental dam used? A dental dam is a piece of rubber that fits over your mouth to reveal only the tooth being worked on. It prevents any bits of mercury amalgam from getting into your mouth or going down your throat. Does the office test patients on the biocompatibility of dental materials before they are placed in the mouth? You're going to live with these materials a long time and they need to be compatible with your individual body so they don't harm your health. Does the dentist test the fillings for electrical current to determine the order of removal? Metal fillings set up an electrical current in the mouth, and need to be removed in correct order so as not to create a problem for you. If the dentist tells you the procedures above are controversial or unnecessary, it usually means s/he has no experience with them.

Changing fillings can be traumatic, even when all the correct procedures are followed. If you have had amalgam fillings in your mouth a long time, you may experience memories or emotions that go back to the time when those fillings were first placed. The teeth are not simply dormant lumps of bone, but have nerves and blood running through them, connecting them with the rest of your body. To make the process as easy on yourself as possible, do not have fillings removed when you are under a great deal of work or personal stress. Be sure to follow an excellent diet prior to the procedure. Some people even go on a cleanse.

Afterwards, teeth may be tender until the new fillings settle in. Mercury residue may linger in other areas of your body. The dentist, a homeopath or naturopath, or a practitioner at the facility where you were tested on dental materials should be able to tell you how to clear this residue.

If the dentist doesn't have you tested on dental materials to find out which ones are biocompatible with your body, arrange for the testing yourself. Don't accept the dentist's affirmation that a dental material is biocompatible *until it has been tested on you.* Some dentists have testing available in their offices or are connected with testing sites at another location. The testing will be an extra charge, but it is well worth it when you consider that dental materials can be in your mouth for the rest of your life!

The problems from dental materials can be considerable. Dr. Huggins reports these symptoms among patients who suspect they are reacting to dental materials: chronic depression, numbness in extremities, frequent urination, chronic fatigue, cold hands and feet, bloating, short term memory lapses, constipation, tremors, leg cramps, ringing in ears, shortness of breath, heartburn, itching and skin rash, insomnia, chest pain, headaches, and diarrhea.

Having the right dental materials in your mouth can change your life. When I got much of the metal out of my mouth, I went from experiencing daily discomfort and regular minor illnesses to feeling great. Of course, the ideal would be to have no cavities or fillings at all! Maybe in my next life....

For more information read:
Let the Tooth Be Known...Are Your Teeth Making You Sick? What you need to know in order to find a
Biological Dentist by Dawn Ewing RDH, PhD, ND, Holistic Health Alternatives, 1998.
Order from: Holistic Health Alternatives, 1011 Whitestone, Houston, TX 77073.
www./.net/~drdawn

20. FEMININE HYGIENE PRODUCTS.

The same problems associated with perfumed products apply to tampons, except this time you're putting the chemicals right inside your body, against tissues which can quickly and easily absorb them into the bloodstream. Scented tampons and other feminine hygiene products are liable to contain formaldehyde, an irritant, mutagen, possible carcinogen, and a trigger of brain and organ dysfunctions.

Most brands of tampons and pads, scented or unscented, contain chlorine bleached fibers. Chlorine is a severe irritant. Synthetic fibers in tampons encourage the growth of bacteria involved in toxic shock syndrome, while cotton fibers have the opposite effect.

I can't help wondering if these chemical laden products contribute to the cramps and other physical, emotional, and mental (fuzzy-brain) symptoms many women feel during their menses. Since our reproductive organs are already doing some of the work of eliminating toxins from our systems, it seems unfair to burden them with additional chemicals.

Once I switched to unbleached cotton tampons and pads, I stopped having cramps. Other women who have switched to unbleached 100% cotton tampons, made some dietary changes, and cleared their homes of toxins tell me they experience no PMS and their periods are pain-free and easy.

Teenaged girls who are starting to use tampons and pads should be encouraged to maintain the health of their reproductive organs by using unscented, all-cotton brands. Tampax advertizes their Original Regular Tampons as all-cotton. At the natural foods store, look for Ecofem, terra femme, Natracare, and Organic Tampons from Eco Yarn. These four brands are 100% cotton, free of chlorine bleach, sterile, and biodegradable. Eco Yarn tampons are also pesticide-free, made from certified organic cotton grown in Texas.

LAUNDRY & CLOTHING

21. TROUBLE IN THE LAUNDRY ROOM.

Laundry products affect your body on a daily basis. Think of it this way. Even after the rinse cycle, detergent and fabric softener leave their residue in your clothes, sheets, and towels. You wear your clothes against your skin all day and you sleep in your sheets all night. So whatever laundry products you use, your body is surrounded by them *24 hours a day*. When those products contain harmful chemicals, your body never has a break from them and, after a while, your health will suffer.

Most conventional laundry products tend to contain toxins. Because these products are so widely available, it's easy to assume they are safe, however, Debra Lynn Dadd points out that *detergent causes more household poisonings than any other product* (most often with children who eat the stuff)! And once you wash your clothes with detergent, it goes into the water system, so you end up drinking it. Detergent ingredients can include suspected carcinogens such as phenol, which impairs digestion and the absorption of protein, ammonia, which irritates mucous membranes and skin, and ethanol which depresses the nervous system, interferes with motor coordination and can cause vertigo, nausea, shock, and hypothermia!

Detergent, fabric softener, and bleach are powerful chemicals. When there are chemical and synthetic scent residues in your clothes, your body may give you any of these signals: chronic cough, eye irritation and skin rashes, digestive and menstrual trouble, breathing problems, fatigue, depression, disorientation, and emotional and behavioral reactions.

Are unscented products easier on your health? To some extent. But fabric softener, according to Balch and Balch, in *Prescription for Nutritional Healing,* contains mercury, a poison which may alter your state considerably. Behavioral reactions to fabric softener can include temper tantrums, weepiness, depression, or feeling spaced out or lethargic—the neurotoxic effect varies depending on genetic and individual makeup. Some people may experience tiredness, headaches, menstrual problems, skin problems, or insomnia. Quite often, the people who react *worst* to fabric softener are also the ones who are most hooked on it!

It's common to crave the very substance that causes your body to do the most masking. Masking is when the body uses up huge supplies of nutrients and enzymes to eliminate toxins and make it look as though nothing is wrong.

Both detergent and fabric softener were invented for synthetic fabrics only. So they are unnecessary for garments and bedding made from natural fibers.

Bleach containing chlorine is another toxic chemical often mistaken for a harmless cleaner. Chlorine was used as a chemical weapon in World War I to gas soldiers in the trenches. It is very dangerous. If you mix chlorine with vinegar or ammonia or any product made with ammonia, the fumes will kill you. Literally. *Bleach must be disposed of at the toxic waste facility.*

Well, now that you know how to conduct chemical warfare with your laundry products, you might decide to get rid of these toxic chemicals. Take them to the toxic waste facility. If you can't bring yourself to throw away your current box of detergent, give it away or finish it and move on to new products that support your health. Whether or not you immediately throw out your detergent, *definitely stop using fabric softener* or switch to a natural one. (see chapter on fabric softeners.) You'll be surprised at the beneficial changes that occur.

When you eliminate these toxins from your life, you could go through some detoxification, involving headaches, tiredness, or other odd symptoms. You might even feel like you have a cold for a couple of days. If this happens, don't be alarmed. Your body is clearing out the chemicals it has been masking, which may involve some minor discomfort. Drink lots of pure water and rest if necessary. It will pass.

22. HEALTH-SUPPORTING LAUNDRY PRODUCTS.

What's your definition of clean? Is the scent of your laundry detergent or fabric softener part of that definition? Advertisers have convinced us that clean smells like lemon or pine or chlorine bleach, but in fact, clean clothes have *no odor* at all, either pleasant or unpleasant. Laundry that is *really* clean contains no artificial scents and no chemical residues from powerful synthetic products. It is simply the clothing minus soil and odors. No additives.

Health-supporting laundry products include natural-source cleaners, liquid soap, washing soda, borax, and white vinegar available at grocery stores or natural products stores. Liquid soap or cleaner works for all your laundry, accompanied by borax for freshening and washing soda for cutting grease and whitening. Nature Clean sells unscented natural-source laundry powder or liquid. Ecover, too, has excellent products, scented from plant sources. Orange Apeel, made from oranges, is useful for removing odors—even skunk!—from clothes and other washables, as well as many other cleaning jobs.

The laundry product that is easiest on clothes and health is laundry discs. Laundry discs are small padded discs filled with ceramic beads. The beads are charged so they create a change in the molecular structure of the water, enabling it to wash the soil from your clothes. Detergents also alter (destabilize) the water molecules but through chemical means. This destabilization helps the water do a better job of cleaning—yes, you heard me right. It's not laundry discs or detergent that actually clean your clothes, it's water!

The initial price of the discs may seem high—$50 as of this writing—but they last for 700 to 750 washes. To do the equivalent amount of laundry with detergent over the same time period would cost you between five and fifteen times as much, or between $250 and $750.

Not only are laundry discs inexpensive, they are terrific for colored clothes and do not dull blacks the way detergent does. Detergent contains bleaching agents, which is why your blacks whiten at the seams and turn charcoal grey. According to Teldon Limited, who market Ecosave products, laundry discs also kill common infection-causing germs, namely E. coli and Staphylococcus aureus.

On the other hand, laundry discs will not brighten your whites. Borax or washing soda does a better job of this. For food or grease marks, rub the spot with a few drops of grease-cutting dish soap as a stain remover before putting into the regular wash. If you still hesitate to give up your detergent, at least select an *unscented* product such as President's Choice Unscented.

Once you choose laundry products that are easy on your body and do not outgas chemical fumes into your home air, your immune system will strengthen and your indoor environment will be fresh and safe for living.

23. NATURAL FABRIC SOFTENER.

Eliminating fabric softener from your life is a good place to start if you want long-term health and a safe and healthy home environment. Clothing that has been fabric-softened keeps you in a day-long cloud of chemicals, synthetic scent, and mercury, with physical and neurotoxic consequences. Fabric softener includes both the liquid you use in the washing machine and the tear-off sheets you put in the dryer.

Fabric softener was developed originally to eliminate static cling, which occurs mainly with synthetic fabrics. Natural fibers do not have this problem. Fabric softener works by coating fabric fibers with chemical which does not wash out. (Similar to the principle of wrinkle-proofing.)

The safest fabric softener is no fabric softener at all. Or use between one half to one cup of vinegar in the final rinse water. Vinegar is easy, inexpensive, and useful for other household chores and has the decided advantage of being perfume- and chemical-free. Some natural foods and earth-wise products stores sell biodegradable fabric softeners. Read labels to be sure they are fragrance-free or scented naturally, not chemically. If you use fabric softener because you like a little scent in your clothes, a non-toxic alternative is to use herbs. Simply tie the herbs you like into a lightweight sock or a square of cheesecloth and put it into the dryer with the clothes. Or, if you like citrus, add a few drops of Orange Apeel to your wash water.

To get the chemicals from fabric softener out of your clothes and bed linens, you will probably need to wash them several times. If you have been using fabric softener sheets, you can sponge the residue from the inside of the dryer with a mixture of baking soda and unscented detergent or cleanser. This may take several washings.

When you buy a new washer or dryer, be sure to tell the salesperson that you do *not* want any fabric softeners in your new machine. Some manufacturers put complimentary bottles or boxes of fabric softener into the appliance before shipping. The perfume and chemicals have lots of time to outgas and coat the inside of the machine before it arrives at your home. Inform your retailer that you will not accept delivery if there is fabric softener in your new appliance.

If your clothes have some electric charge, you are probably overdrying them. Try cutting back on the drying time, or use a spray bottle to mist your clothes with water if they are too dry. A light spritz of water will eliminate static charge without making dry clothes too wet to wear. You might also consider hanging your clothes on a line to dry naturally. In the winter, I hang damp clothes on hangers and hook them over any convenient doorframe inside the house as an impromptu indoor clothesline. While the clothes are drying, they help humidify the air.

One reason washed clothes are stiff is because of your detergent! Laundry detergent tends to stick in the clothes, leaving chemical and perfume residues that harden the fabric. I noticed how much stiffer detergent-washed clothes were after I started using laundry discs. My clothes came out of the dryer softer than they did with any other laundry product. There is more to this than my imagination. Teldon Limited says that dissolved lime in the wash water usually re-crystallizes on the laundry (and your washing machine), but with the discs, it is unable to do so. Instead, it drains away with the waste water after a load of washing. So, the safest laundry product for your health also gives you the softest clothes!

If you have trouble parting with your fabric softener, you're in good company. There are strong external and internal pressures to use it and you will need some powerful self-love to overcome those influences. It's well worth it!

24. STAIN REMOVAL WITHOUT TEARS.

Chlorine bleach has been the classic stain remover for whites, however, it is a severe lung irritant, harms all mucous membranes on the way to the lungs, and is implicated in circulatory problems and diabetes. Chlorine and its fumes, either from bleach or from chlorinated tap or swimming pool water, can bring on skin rashes, dizzy spells, and digestive disorders, and is a risk factor in cancers of the gastrointestinal and urinary tracts.

Non-chlorine bleaches that biodegrade to oxygen are safer, or you can use hydrogen peroxide. If you've been using bleach on germs or mold, you can use hydrogen peroxide for the same purpose. Laundry discs kill germs, and direct (outdoor) hot sunshine will help kill mold. (see chapter on Mold for other solutions)

Here is a short list of non-toxic home treatments for stains. Treat stains as quickly as possible before they have a chance to set into your clothing. Wash clothing as usual after treating for stains.

• *Blood:* If you can get to it right away, pour salt or cold water on the stain. Soak in cold water. Wash with cold water and soap. For stubborn stains, try a mixture of borax and water (four tablespoons of borax in two cups water) for white fabrics. For colors, mix cornstarch with cornmeal in water to make a soggy paste. Let mixture dry on the stain, then brush off.

• *Caffeines* (chocolate, coffee): Rub stain with cold water then with borax and water (one to two tablespoons in two cups water). OR Rub stain with a mixture of egg yolk and lukewarm water. OR Use dish soap on the spot.

• *Diapers:* Soak in a bucket or basin in warm water mixed with four tablespoons baking soda. To disinfect, add a half teaspoon or five drops tea tree oil (available at natural foods stores) or wash with laundry discs. OR Soak in diluted Orange Apeel. Wash in hot water. OR Soak in water and accelerated hydrogen peroxide (Virox).

- **Fruit/Juice:** Pour boiling water over the stain. OR Cold soda water or salt can be poured on the stain immediately. Soak in milk. (Milk must be rinsed out with cold water only.)
- **Gum:** Rub gum with ice so it flakes off.
- **Grass:** Rub stain with glycerin soap, then let it set for an hour before washing.
- **Food stains:** The best all-purpose stain remover for food or grease marks is a few drops of grease-cutting dish liquid such as Soap Factory or Ecover.
- **Grease:** Baking soda and washing soda are good grease cutters. For whites: Pour boiling water over the stain and rub with baking or washing soda. For colors: Wet stain with warm water, then use a few drops of grease-cutting dish soap and rub.

If you get grease on a nice silk garment, here's a tip I learned in a clothing store: Lay the garment out. Now, cover the stain with dry corn starch and leave it to sit overnight. The cornstarch lifts the grease out of the fabric. *Do not wet the fabric or the corn starch.* The following day, brush off the cornstarch. The stain should be gone. If not, leave a while longer. If the garment needs washing, wash it only after brushing away all the cornstarch. I have tried this and it works! I have also found cornstarch lifts out grease marks on upsholstery.

- **Ink:** Soak in cold water. OR Soak in milk. (Rinse milk out with cold water.) OR Treat stain with hydrogen peroxide.
- **Milk:** Soak in cool water. OR Soak in warm water and treat with glycerin soap.
- **Urine:** Rub with baking soda dissolved in water. Rinse in warm water. OR Use diluted Orange Apeel.

If you or your family members are stain-prone, you may want to consider avoiding white and pale solid color clothing.

25. SIMPLE WAYS YOUR CLOTHES CAN SUPPORT YOUR HEALTH.

I used to wear a down-filled parka in the winter when I took my dog for his walk. I'd arrive home exhausted, wondering why I felt lousy after an outing that was supposed to make me feel healthy! I had a similar reaction on rainy days in spring when I wore a plastic raincoat.

For a long time I blamed myself, thinking I just wasn't in very good shape. Then, one day, I found out I reacted to feathers and plastic. I switched to a wool coat and an umbrella and suddenly I could walk for hours without tiring. In fact, the dog became the one who wanted to go home and rest!

This was a big lesson in how powerfully clothing can affect the body and its energy level. As many people do, I felt tired and uncomfortable wearing synthetics such as polyester and acrylic, made from petrochemicals. In general, the most health-supporting fibers are cotton, linen, silk, hemp, rayon, ramie, and wool.

Your clothing can expose you to chemicals through fiber content, dyes, pesticides, and cleaning methods. To avoid these hazards, buy natural fibers and avoid heavy dyes, fabric softener, and perchloroethylene dry cleaning—a highly toxic process. GreenEarth dry cleaners use a health-safe silicone process. To locate one near you, visit www.greenearthcleaning.com. Launder new clothing before wearing to wash out any sizing or lingering pesticides. When you are giving your children clothing as a gift (e.g. new pajamas at Christmas), launder before gift-wrapping, since children tend to try on and wear new clothes immediately.

Natural fiber underwear is particularly important. Nylon and too-tight underwear are known to encourage local infection and irritation for both men and women.

Bras have been associated with breast cancer by some researchers. Breast cancer incidence is said to be highest among women who wear their bras for the greatest number of hours. Perhaps this is because where the bra presses tightly against the body, it obstructs the movement of lymphatic fluid. The lymph is part of the immune system and helps to carry away toxins, but when the lymph can't move because an elastic or wire is pressing against it, the toxins just sit there in the chest area. Yuck.

You may decide to wear a bra only when necessary. If you work out of your home, you may not have to wear one very often. If you need to wear a bra to work, make sure you take it off when you get home and leave it off on weekends when relaxing. *Never* wear your bra to bed (yes, believe it or not, people *do* this!). Look for a natural fiber bra—cotton, silk—that is free from bones, wires and push-up type structuring. Women who do not absolutely need to wear a bra may prefer cotton or silk camisoles.

Once you've cleared the chemical toxins out of your life, you may notice you feel less than terrific after a few hours in the shopping mall. Malls are full of outgassing plastics, scents, and chemicals in the new products and shopping bags, and have poor air circulation. If you're looking at clothes in a big mall, you may want to keep your shopping time—and your exposure to the toxins in that environment—to a minimum. People who are quite chemically sensitive may feel better shopping in smaller stores that open directly to the outdoors and have a lower concentration of toxic materials in their interiors.

Keep dirty laundry anywhere but the bedroom, especially if you work with petrochemicals or smoke, otherwise you will breath in fumes and pollutants from your clothes all night. During pollen season, if you are pollen sensitive, avoid hanging your clothes outside on a clothesline to dry as they will be coated with pollen by the time you bring them in. To protect yourself from wearing pollen-coated clothing, allow clothes to dry indoors during the spring.

A final clothing suggestion: wear flat shoes. High heels and varying heel heights can cause foot and back problems with potential degenerative carry-over in later life.

HOME REMEDIES

Warning: This chapter is not intended to be prescriptive nor is it a replacement for medical advice and attention. Do not rely on remedies in the case of trauma such as broken bone, animal bite, poisoning, or other serious accident or medical emergency. Seek immediate medical attention for any traumatic condition. Refer to a physician for any health concern.

26. ADDITIONS TO THE MEDICINE CABINET.

What's in *your* medicine cabinet? Whatever the contents, they will reflect your typical symptoms and give you an excellent idea of where you may need to make changes in your life.

For every chronic symptom I had, whether it was a runny nose, indigestion or headache, medication provided temporary relief, but did not solve my underlying problem. Instead, my symptoms went away when I eliminated poorly-tolerated foods and chemicals, improved my indoor environment and my drinking water, and got more exercise. Since making these changes, I haven't needed an over-the-counter or prescription medication in years.

If I *did* need to, of course, I would utilize conventional medicine. As Dr. Bruce Pomeranz puts it, save the penicillin for the times when you *really* need it, for example, if you develop pneumococcal pneumonia. When life is not at stake, he suggests, there are many other resources and methods to use for well-being.

Kathy and I both keep certain home remedies on hand for occasions when they may be helpful. Here is a list:

• **Acidophilus** is an anti-fungal usually taken by mouth. For women, there's another way to use it. If you have a yeast infection, acidophilus is very effective at restoring the natural environment of the vagina, according to a doctor I spoke to at a gynecological clinic. In her opinion, acidophilus is just as effective as the typical medications she prescribes—and far less expensive.

Her advice was to insert one capsule of acidophilus at bedtime every night for a week. You can wear a pad if concerned about leakage. By the end of the week, the yeast infection should be gone. If not, continue as necessary. Women who've tried this tell me their infections have cleared within the week.

If you are dairy-sensitive like me, look for a brand of acidophilus that is made from a different source. Kyodophilus is potato-based, and there is also a carrot-based acidophilus on the market. Ask in your natural foods or supplements store.

• *Arnica montana* is a homeopathic remedy available in drops or tablets. If you have bruising from an injury, have overstressed your muscles or have had a tooth pulled with subsequent trauma to the surrounding tissue, Arnica can help.

If you are a person who bruises easily and continually, you are probably missing important nutrients. Rather than taking Arnica, increase your level of B and C vitamins, essential fatty acids, and fresh vegetables. Bilberry extract may be helpful. Make sure you are eating adequate protein. Caffeine, sugars, alcohol, and especially smoking contribute to excess bruising because they use up so many of your essential nutrients. Bruising may also be a symptom in some disease conditions. Check with your doctor.

• *Bach Flower Rescue Remedy* is an all-purpose flower essence for distress. You can use it when you have an ache of any kind, or have suffered an upset of a mental, emotional or physical nature. I often use it in combination with Arnica to calm and soothe after a minor mishap such as an accidental cut, bruise or blow. Rescue Remedy comes in drops. It has an alcohol base, so if you're sensitive to alcohol you can put it on your skin rather than ingesting it. The crook of the elbow or the skin on either side of the navel are good spots to put the drops. Let them sit for five or ten seconds before rubbing into your skin.

You can use Arnica and Rescue Remedy on your pet by gently rubbing two or three drops into the skin just inside the ear where the fur is thin or non-existent. If it's easier, put some in a little water for the pet to drink or squirt directly onto the pet's tongue. (However, use remedies for minor mishaps only. Always check with your veterinarian if your pet is injured.)

• *Enzymes* help with digestion. As you age, you use up your body's supply of enzymes, so outside help comes in handy. Taking enzymes before a meal will help prevent gas, bloating, and indigestion, particularly if you eat a food that doesn't agree with you well or contains lots of indigestible fiber, like beans. You can also take enzymes to help eliminate cold viruses. (see chapter on Frequent Colds.)

Some brands of enzyme we like are Udo's Choice Ultimate Enzyme Blend, Nu-Life's Dyna-Gest Ultra-zyme, and papaya enzymes. Any broad-spectrum natural source enzyme designed to digest proteins, lipids (fats), and carbohydrates will do the trick. Buy at your natural foods store.

• *Ginger root* is a powerful anti-inflammatory agent, according to Andrew Weil, M.D. I find it works well for injuries, muscle pain, and arthritic-type stiffness. If you like the taste, it can be eaten raw or cooked, pickled or candied, or you can buy it in capsules at the natural foods store. Ginger has anti-nauseant properties so you can use it to combat travel sickness or seasickness. It is also considered an aid to digestion.

Stephen Fulder, Ph.D., calls ginger "the ultimate home remedy". In addition to its anti-inflammatory and anti-nauseant qualities, ginger is good for the liver, and has antibiotic, antihistamine, analgesic, anti-fungal, muscle relaxant, anti-viral, and antiseptic properties. It may also lower fever, stimulate circulation, and discourage insects.

• *Milk Thistle* is an herb available in capsules in natural foods stores. Milk thistle helps the liver function well to clear toxins. It's great for city dwellers who go to work in a polluted downtown environment, anyone who commutes in rush hour traffic, and for those times when you celebrate with rich, heavy foods or a few too many glasses of wine. Considering our polluted global environment and the fact that the liver does the lion's share of clearing toxins, milk thistle is helpful any time, particularly when you are under stress.

• *Olbas pastilles and Olbas oil* are great for colds and coughs. The pastilles help to soothe your sore throat, and the oil can be used to open up stuffy nasal passages. Olbas oil can also be used on stiff muscles. Look for these products in the natural foods store.

- **Tea tree oil** is a terrific all-around disinfectant and topical antifungal. We have used it on athlete's foot, as a mouth rinse for sore gums, and as a skin disinfectant. I've also used it in my dog's ears in the summer when he gets a yeasty overgrowth from swimming.
- **Vitamin E** can be used directly on a cut. Break open a capsule and smear it on the cut. This may help prevent scarring. Apply similarly to very chapped lips as a healing gloss.

If the skin on your fingers or hands tends to dry out and split open in winter, squeeze vitamin E from a capsule onto the split spots and cover loosely with adhesive strips for about 24 hours. During this time, the skin will start to reform and seal instead of splitting open again. You can then remove the adhesive strips and allow the splits to heal in the open air.

27. TIRED? TRY THIS.

- **Drink water.** You may be dehydrated. When you're thirsty, your body can react with tiredness, because water is important to so many physical functions including brain activity. Other liquids will not help since they are processed as food. Coffee, regular tea, chocolate drinks, soft drinks, and alcohol won't work to rehydrate you since they all have a *de*hydrating effect.
- **Breathe deeply and/or exercise**, even if it is only to get up out of your chair and stretch or walk around a little. Make a concious effort to take a few deep breaths and exhale completely. If you've been sitting for some time working, reading or watching t.v., your breathing shallows, robbing your body of sufficient oxygen. I always feel best on the days when I've been for a two or three hour hike, inhaling lots of fresh air and working my muscles.
- **Check for allergies and sensitivities.** Notice if you are tired after meals— you may be reacting to foods, particularly grains. Chemical overload is another possibility.
- **Are you more tired in winter?** Your heating system may be at fault—

nitrogen dioxide in natural gas reduces the blood's capacity to transport oxygen. Or you may need to clear other toxins and chemicals from your indoor environment and personal care products. In winter, when you spend more time indoors with windows closed, you will be more affected by these toxins than at other seasons.

• *Are you more tired in spring and fall?* Find out if you are reacting to pollen or mold in the air. Either of these stresses to the immune system can be tiring.

• *Cut back on wheat, dairy, and grains.* Wheat, corn, sugar, and other grains are among the most common food allergens and may be exhausting you as your immune and digestive systems struggle to process them.

• *Take enzymes and essential fatty acids* provided by products such as Ultimate Enzyme Blend, Ultra-zyme, Udo's Choice Oil Blend, or hemp oil. I find when my body is well supplied with the enzymes and EFAs it needs, I have much more energy, need less sleep, and rarely feel tired during the day.

• *Cut out cooked and poor quality fats and oils.* Excess dietary fat can make you sluggish. Inferior quality fats and oils are especially hard on you since they tend to be loaded with chemicals and are so overcooked your body can no longer recognize them as anything but toxins (and the more toxins you have to process, the more tired you'll be.)

• *Eat regular meals that contain protein.* There was a time when I expected myself to function all day on a quart of coffee and a muffin. For part of the day, I'd fly high but by about 4 p.m., I crashed and was very tired. *And* crabby. Now, I eat regular meals of *real* food, like fruits, veggies, whole grains, nuts, soy products, eggs, fish, and chicken. I don't eat all these foods at every meal, but I do eat small amounts of protein over the course of the day and it's paid big dividends in terms of my energy level.

• *Support your adrenal glands.* Modern life is stressful and stimulates adrenaline output, so adrenals need lots of support. Feed your adrenals with vitamin B-12, pantothenic acid (B-5) and folic acid. According to wellness consultant, David Slater, wild cherry and licorice root also nourish the adrenals.

In *What Your Doctor May Not Tell You About Premenopause,* John R. Lee, M.D., points out that overworked adrenals can result in blood sugar problems and excess weight, as well as muscle and memory loss. To restore the adrenals, he recommends lots of rest and restful activities such as gardening, playing a musical instrument or spending time with your pet.

• *Check your emotional state.* Tiredness can be related to depression, and depression can be related to low levels of serotonin. Serotonin is the calming neurotransmitter.

To boost it, build up your supply of amino acids over the day by eating some protein at every meal. Then, to stimulate serotonin production, eat a plain carbohydrate such as a potato, apple, carrot, small glass of juice, bowl of popcorn or cereal, three hours after dinner or just before you go to bed. Do not eat any protein with this carbohydrate (so no milk with the cereal, no cheese on the potato or popcorn—butter or oil is fine, no peanut butter or nuts with the apple).

Of course, chemistry is not the only reason for depression, but getting your brain chemistry under control will aid you significantly in dealing with your emotional state. For more information, read *Potatoes Not Prozac* by Kathleen DesMaisons, Ph.D. and *Natural Prozac* by Joel Robertson, M.D.

Deepak Chopra, Joan Borysenko, and other doctors and researchers recommend meditation as a means to combat depression, de-stress, and enable better sleep.

• *Sleep more.* This may sound obvious, but many, many people are sleep-deprived and have unrealistic expectations of how their bodies ought to perform. Has our performance-crazed culture given you the message that sleeping is a weakness? Don't believe it! Many accidents with dangerous or tragic consequences occur because workers and professionals are sleep-deprived. Tired people drive as poorly as those who are alcohol-impaired.

Sleeping eight or nine hours a night is normal, not excessive. Before the advent of electric light, people slept an average of nine and a half hours a night. And if you are under stress, you need *more* sleep than usual, not less.

As the Zen saying goes: When hungry, eat. When tired, sleep.

28. FREQUENT COLDS? TRY THIS.

• *When you feel a cold coming on, take digestive enzymes.* This technique is recommended by Udo Erasmus, Ph.D., who explains cold viruses have a protein coating. The enzyme digests the coating, leaving the virus without protection so it dies. Enzymes also free the immune system from involvement with digestion so it can spend more time chasing down virus. Digestion uses more of your body's resources than any other process. (Hence the old saying, "If you feed a cold, you will have to starve a fever.")

Dr. Erasmus suggests you take enzymes consistently over the course of the day if you are coming down with a cold, and take three or four before you go to sleep. I have done this and found it extremely effective. (I take three or four about four hours apart, but you could also spread them out and take one every hour or two.)

• *Stay off sweets.* Sugars slow down immune function significantly for up to five hours after you eat them. If you're a big sugar eater and catch colds often, try going off sweets completely. If that's too much of a wrench, upgrade your sweets to fruit-juice or rice-syrup sweetened cookies, cakes, and frozen desserts available in the natural foods store. The lower sugar content will be easier on your immune system while satisfying your sweet tooth. (*Cookbooks* listed after Resource Guide contain sugarless dessert recipes.)

• *Eat more vegetables.* Vegetables are full of vitamins, minerals, and fiber, and help to clear some toxins from the body, making it easier to resist invaders like cold viruses.

• *Raise your total immune picture.* Since making the changes we recommend in this book, Kathy and I have both found we rarely get sick or contract a cold, even when "everybody" has it.

• *Sleep and rest.* Sometimes immunity is low because you haven't had enough sleep or are going through a stressful time. Try to get enough rest, especially during times of stress, even if it means cutting back on other activities. North Americans are probably more sleep-deprived than any other group, and there are serious health and safety consequences.

• *Laugh and have fun.* Laughter definitely stimulates the immune system. Leading neuropeptide researcher, Candace Pert, Ph.D., points out that your emotions and immune system are linked through chemical messengers in your body, so things that make you feel great emotionally will do the same for you on the physical level.

• *Spend time with people you love.* In *Love and Survival,* Dean Ornish, M.D., demonstrates that loving and supportive relationships may be more important to health than any other single factor, despite the undeniable value of healthful physical habits.

29. TROUBLE SLEEPING? TRY THIS.

• *Are you ingesting too much caffeine before bed?* Check on how much chocolate, coffee, regular tea, carbonated beverage, and alcohol you consume late in the day. All these items speed up your heart rate and may keep you awake.

• *Are you overstimulating your brain with news, violent or exciting television shows, movies or books before you go to bed?* As author and lecturer Jack Canfield explains, while you sleep, your brain replays whatever you watch or read during the evening. If the material is violent or disturbing, like the evening news or a horror movie, your sleep may be disturbed by repeat mental performances. Try soft music, comedy, a good book, prayer, meditation or quiet time instead. Your whole system needs to gear down in the evening before going to bed.

• *Are you giving yourself enough time to sleep?* The amount of sleep you think your body needs is dictated as much by the culture we live in as by actual need. In the pre-industrial world, people slept an average of nine and a half hours a night. Today, we think a few short hours is enough, despite heightened demands on our nervous systems. If you're not allowing your body enough time to get a good night's rest, you may be in a state of hyperviligance, unable to relax completely because you expect to have to jump out of bed at any minute. Try going to bed a little earlier. Experiment with the number of sleep hours that make you feel really good.

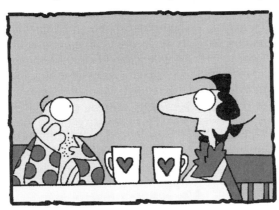

"I had 25 cups of coffee this morning
before I finally realized you bought decaf."

• *Is your bedroom dark enough?* The eyes need full darkness to relax completely. If there is too much light in your bedroom from outdoor or indoor sources, it may be keeping you awake. Make sure your curtains or blinds provide a "black-out" from streetlights and other ambient outside light.

• *Trouble sleeping can be due to chemicals in the bedroom.* If your system is having to work hard all night to maintain homeostasis in a toxic bedroom environment, you will not have a good sleep or be able to relax fully. Your body needs its sleep time for healing, rest, and repair work. The next few suggestions have to do with creating a health-supporting bedroom environment.

• *Are you storing piles of newspapers, magazines, and books next to your bed?* Printed material outgasses chemicals, especially if it's new. Old books can be moldy. Reading material that sits around for some time collects dust.

For the best sleep, keep your printed material outside the bedroom, except for the one or two items you are currently reading. If you have drawers in your bedside table, keep the items there when not in use, especially while you're sleeping. When my husband and I liberated our bedroom from our stacks of books and magazines, there was a significant change in the quality of our bedroom air and I definitely slept better.

• *Is your bedroom full of scented products?* Because of the hundreds of possible chemical combinations in perfumed and scented products, if you have them in your bedroom, you're sleeping in a toxic swamp. Check for scented candles, drawer liners, pot pourri, room deodorants, sachets (home-made herbal sachets are okay), hangers, cosmetics, and personal care products.

• *Do you have candles in your bedroom?* If the candles are paraffin, not beeswax, corn or soybean oil, you're breathing in petrochemicals all night. Store them in a tin or large glass jar.

• *Check your bedding and sleepwear.* Are you reacting to feathers, down, synthetic fabrics, fireproofed or stainproofed bed coverings, fabric softener or scented detergent in sheets and pillowslips, the petrochemical cover on your waterbed, or the electrical field of your waterbed or electric blanket? Any of these can cause sleep problems.

I used to adore down pillows until I found out they were the reason I couldn't get out of bed in the morning. Once I changed to a polyester-stuffed pillow, my sleep time went from 12 hours to 7 or 8. (I know, I know, polyester is a petrochemical but, for some reason, I don't react to the foam inside my pillow—perhaps because it is a "dormant" petrochemical, no pun intended, unlike the ones that get inside the body through food, cosmetics, outgassing, etc. Also, you can wash your polyester pillow in the washing machine to remove any chemicals in the fabric covering.) Or you might prefer a pillow stuffed with buckwheat hulls, available in Oriental stores, bedding shops or by mail order from Gaiam. Wool batting-stuffed pillows are also very comfy.

For better rest, try washing your pillow and/or putting it outside in full sunlight for several hours. Dust mites build up every four to five weeks and may be affecting your sleep pattern. If you feel stuffed-up, have twitchy legs, cough or have other allergic-type symptoms but feel better a few minutes after you leave your bed, dust mites may be the problem.

• **Is your furniture outgassing formaldehyde?** If you have bedroom furniture made with particle board, seal it with wood sealer to prevent formaldehyde outgassing into your bedroom air for years and years. In particular, seal the backs of dressers and shelving units and the undersides of drawers where particle- and press-board tends to be completely exposed. Also check baby cribs, bunk beds, and children's captain beds (beds with built-in drawers underneath.)

• **Is your bedroom carpeted?** Carpet is full of toxins including dust mites, bacteria, mold, and chemicals. Hardwood or ceramic tile is a better choice, with a small, washable, cotton throw rug beside the bed if you like to step out of bed onto fabric.

• **Did you recently paint or renovate your bedroom?** Unless you have used all natural and safe materials, toxic fumes may still be outgassing into your bedroom air from paint, wallpaper, curtains, bedcoverings or furniture.

Try sleeping elsewhere for a week while you try one of the following: take living creatures (plants, pets) out of the room, close bedroom windows and doors to seal the room, turn up the heat and let the toxins cook out of the new materials in your bedroom for several hours or, if possible, a full day. If your bedroom is the only room that has been renovated, put a damp, rolled-up towel at the bottom of the door to keep the toxins from leaking out into the rest of your house. If several rooms or your whole house has been renovated, close the windows, leave the interior doors open, and *go somewhere else* while the heat is up. Make sure to take your pets with you.

After a few hours, come back and turn off the heat. But don't move back in yet! The household air will be *filled* with toxins. Quickly open all the windows for at least half an hour to allow the toxins to blow away before you spend time indoors again. In particular, children, pets, pregnant women, and anyone with compromised immunity should not be allowed back in until the toxins have dissipated.

If the heat method doesn't appeal to you, try an air filter machine. Let the machine run in your bedroom with the door closed for at least 24 hours, while you sleep elsewhere. Stay out for a week and run the machine several hours every day. This is slower than the heat method, so you may require the air filter machine even after you move back in, at least for a few weeks.

• And finally, **try taking calcium in some form before bed**. Increasing your level of serotonin will also help, since serotonin is the calming brain chemical and the higher your level, the more relaxed you will be. See *Tired? Try this.* for information on raising serotonin levels through diet. Other methods include aerobic exercise, meditation, prayer, listening to calming music or waves on the beach, walking in nature, and writing in a journal.

30. CONSTIPATED? TRY THIS.

• *Drink water.* Dehydration is a major cause of constipation. Choose filtered or distilled water—chemicals in regular tap water, especially chlorine, may affect your bowel function. Avoid caffeine, since it will only dehydrate you further. To alleviate constipation quickly, *Prescription for Nutritional Healing* recommends drinking a glass of water every ten minutes for 30 minutes.

• *Eat more veggies.* The bowel needs lots of roughage to keep things moving through it and fresh vegetables are the best source. Fruit's good too. Try to eat organically-grown versions, since chemicals may affect bowel function.

• *Stay off flour products.* Have you ever made glue from white flour and water? Whenever you eat a food made with white flour, you might as well be filling your intestines with glue. Flour products include bread, bagels, cake, cookies, crackers, muffins, pasta, hot dog and hamburger rolls, some cereals, some types of potato chips, gravies, and sauces.

• *Take enzymes.* Enzymes will help your food to digest better.

• *Choose top quality oils.* Digestive and excretory functions require essential fatty acids which are processed out of most foods. Udo's Oil Blend, hemp seed oil, and pumpkin seed oil contain high levels of essential fatty acids and are some of the best choices for improving bowel function. When buying the last two oils, be sure they are top-quality and properly processed, otherwise you may be ingesting a rancid or chemically-treated product. EFA ratios vary from oil to oil.

Avoid fried and deep-fried foods, since they are almost impossible to digest.

• *Take freshly ground flax seeds.* Udo Erasmus reports the mucilage and fiber in flax seeds alleviate constipation within three days. Drink lots of water to assist the flushing out process. Flax seeds can be ground with a mortar and pestle or in a coffee bean grinder.

• *Cut back on meat consumption.* Vegetables and fruit transit through the intestines in a few hours while meat can take several days! If you are a regular meat eater, try reducing quantities until you are no longer constipated, and eat lots of veggies with your meat to speed up its transit time.

• *Move!* Moving the body helps the bowels to move. Jumping on a mini-trampoline is especially helpful, but any kind of movement will do: walking, dancing, skiing, cycling, swimming, skateboarding, yoga, whatever you like best.

If you are ill, or unable to move much due to injury, arrange pillows on a bed or couch so you can lie on a slant, with your rear and legs higher than your head and shoulders. Now, tap or massage gently along your lower abdomen over your intestines. Start on the right, just above the point where your leg joins your abdomen, a few inches in from your hip bone. Go up the right side of your belly to just below the navel, then across to the left, then down the left side. Cross to the right, just above your pubic bone and begin again. Repeat several times.

The reason for inverting your posture and for tapping or massaging up on the right is because your intestines actually go up and across before they go down again. This process will stimulate movement in your intestines. (It can also stimulate the passage of gas, so you may not want to do it in a room full of people!)

• *Eat prunes.* It's an old remedy, but a good one. Prunes have lots of fiber and definite laxative qualities. Drink water with them to keep things moving.

• *Avoid chemical toxins and poorly tolerated foods.* Foods and chemicals can shut down your bowel's ability to function. Chlorine, for example, is implicated in bowel problems. Formaldehyde, scented products, and petrochemicals can affect you similarly. This is why it's a good idea to clear your home of chemical products.

The foods that are among the top allergens, such as wheat, corn, dairy, and sugar, can also cause bowel problems, whether constipation or diarrhea. This can be true of any food to which you react badly.

Note: If you are regularly constipated, check with your doctor. Constipation can be a symptom of some disease conditions. If you have diarrhea longer than three days, have a doctor check for virus or parasites. Once this is ruled out, check for food and chemical sensitivities, as these are often the cause of bowel trouble.

31. MENSTRUAL DISCOMFORT? TRY THIS.

• *If you have cramps during your period*, your brand of feminine hygiene products may be the problem. I found when I switched to tampons made from organic cotton, free of chlorine bleach and other chemicals, I no longer had any cramps. Bleach, scent, and chemicals may be upsetting your internal environment. Look for unbleached cotton, unscented pads and tampons in the natural foods or environmental products store.

• Annemarie Colbin, author of *Food and Healing* suggests *foods containing hormones from other species contribute to menstrual irregularities.* Eggs, meat, and dairy foods would be in this group, but dairy in particular may be the problem. Try avoiding these foods for a week before your period and see if you have an improvement. You may wish to stay off dairy permanently if it is causing your menstrual problems, or switch to another form, such as goat or sheep cheese and yogurt.

Hormones in food may contribute to mid-cycle cramps, around ovulation time.

• *Other food culprits* include caffeine, sugar, wheat, alcohol, and processed or cooked fats. In the bad old days, when I used to eat lots of chocolate bars (containing caffeine, wheat, and lots of sugar), my cramps were so bad, I once had to go to the hospital! Nothing is more embarrassing and aggravating than to have an emergency room doctor tell you, "There's nothing wrong with you. It's just cramps." *He* should have such cramps before deciding they're "nothing".

Of course the poor guy didn't know what was *really* wrong. After a little research, observation, and experimentation, I changed my diet and feminine hygiene products and my cramps disappeared.

One caution about cutting out these foods is that it's easier to do it in the middle of your cycle—about two weeks before your period begins. When you eliminate foods you've been eating regularly, you may experience some detoxing, which can involve tiredness, headaches, depression or crankiness—*not* something you want to go through during your period. Also, detoxing right at period time may increase cramps, since the reproductive system is also a pathway of elimination for toxins.

• *If you must eat chocolate*, as many women do around the time of their periods, buy top-quality, *organically-grown* chocolate, sweetened *without* sugar, from the natural foods store. You can purchase chocolate bars, cocoa powder (to mix with soy, rice or almond drink instead of cow's milk), wheat-free chocolate chip cookies, and frozen chocolate desserts that taste like ice cream but are made from rice or soy. The reason for doing this is to have the chocolate you crave, while avoiding the chemical toxins from pesticides, fertilizers and processing contained in regular chocolate and sugar-sweetened products.

Many organic chocolate products are sweetened with Sucanat or unrefined organically-grown cane juice crystals. This is a superior product to regular sugar since it is chemical- and bleach-free and may contain some residual minerals. However, if you are sensitive to grains such as wheat or corn, cane sugar is from the same botanical family (called Grass Grains), and even the superior unrefined version of sugar may cause problems at period time.

• *If you crave sweets around period time, try eating a protein first.* When your body is craving protein, you may mistake this for sweet-craving. I did this for years, until I started eating some protein at every meal.

Sweet-craving can result from low levels of neurotransmitters. If you're looking for an energy boost or a means of assuaging depression, sweets may come to mind first. However, Dr. Joel Robertson associates menstrual changes and some depression with low levels of norepinephrine, which is increased by eating protein, not sweets.

• *Eat only top quality fats.* As Udo Erasmus puts it, bad fats contribute to "internal pollution" which contributes to menstrual problems.

• *Avoid chemicals.* Many chemicals are hormone disrupters, so they may be disrupting yours during your cycle. Especially avoid plastics, perfumes, and fabric softener which contains mercury, a poison.

• *Have yourself checked for candida.* Candida is a yeast in every body. In some bodies, however, it overgrows especially if you have taken antibiotics or birth control pills, or have a diet high in refined carbohydrates, including alcohol. Too much yeast can contribute to menstrual problems. There are various treatments for candida, including eating a whole foods diet, using homeopathy, acupressure and desensitization, and taking antifungals. A wellness consultant or natural health care provider can test you for candida and recommend solutions.

SHELTER

32. MAKE YOUR HOME A POLLUTION-FREE OASIS.

C linical ecologists tell us no matter how polluted the outdoor air, the environment in the average house is usually far worse! In *Poisoning Our Children*, Nancy Sokol Green cites a 15-year study of death rates from cancer in women. Some remained at home during the day and others worked outside the home. The women at home had a 54% higher death rate from cancer than the outside group! The study attributed this extraordinary difference to the dangerous toxins and chemicals in products regularly used by the homemakers.

While it's a bit discouraging to think you're courting cancer or some other fatal disease every time you clean the house or do the dishes, take heart! Not all products are equally threatening. Lots of safe ones are now available. Even better, safe household products tend to be less expensive than their toxic counterparts. Over the next few chapters, we'll look at these products and the techniques you can use to make your house into a pollution-free, health-supporting haven.

After choosing safe products to put on your skin and in your mouth, the most important step is to clear your house of toxins. You may be surprised to discover your home is full of petrochemicals, formaldehyde, solvents, mold, and poisons, all of which release molecules into your indoor air and add to your total toxic load. Fortunately, you can control the quality of your air and what goes into your body while you're at home by containing, reducing, and eliminating toxic products. If anyone in your house reacts to pet fur or dander, the more you reduce indoor toxins, the less pets are likely to affect that person.

Safe products are vital to the health of your children and pets. Children's immune systems are still developing so they are even more sensitive than adults to the effects of chemicals. Small children, like pets, spend time on the floor where they receive direct exposure to the cleaners, waxes, and carpet deodorizers you use. They put anything, no matter how yucky, into their mouths and are always in danger of poisoning themselves by eating or drinking out of brightly colored containers whose warning labels they can't read. Pets lick surfaces or get products on their skin and fur. While grooming themselves, they receive direct toxic exposure.

Animal observation has shown a definite connection between chemical exposure and genetic mutation. In humans, this may show up as reproductive or other health problems that manifest in current and future generations. (You, your children, and their children.) Over time, the toxic buildup of chemicals in your body contributes to degenerative conditions and disease, keeping your immune system in a constantly stressed-out state.

Once you make your home into a pollution-free oasis, your immune system can spend its time there relaxing and recuperating from the stresses of the day. When your indoor environment is toxin-free, your body will more easily deal with pollutants encountered *outside* the home, and keep you healthy!

Household & Dish Cleaners

33. ARE YOUR CLEANERS SAFE?

Whether you wipe it, spray it or shake it, when you use a cleaner on any surface in your home, the chemicals in it stick there and outgas into your air. In sealed houses with year-round controlled air, toxic fumes from cleaning products circulate constantly, loading your immune system with an endless amount of work.

Furniture oil and polish, silver polish, oven cleaner, floor cleaner, abrasive cleanser, all-purpose liquid, foam and spray products for glass and other surfaces may be labelled with warnings about their short-term effects, but carry *no information about the long-term health problems*. This is no guarantee of safety!

Manufacturers have not been required to provide information about the health effects of their cleaning products or list their ingredients, so it is difficult to learn what toxins they contain. Chlorine, dye, phenol, nitrobenzene, formaldehyde, fragrance, ammonia, ethanol, napthalene, petroleum distillates, and aerosol propellants are some of the possible toxic ingredients. These chemicals have been linked to eye and skin irritation, cancer, heart problems, high blood pressure, hormonal and genetic changes, headaches, dizziness, effects on the nervous system, liver damage, diabetes, and birth defects.

There are two major problems with household cleaners available on the market today: chemicals and scent. Strictly speaking, scent falls into the category of chemicals too, because it's *made* from chemicals. All those products that say "fresh scent" on them are not perfumed by spring flowers or just-picked lemons. The fragrance is produced from hundreds of mostly chemical ingredients and is synthetically fixed, or held, in the cleaner. Formaldehyde is a typical fixative—remember formaldehyde from high school biology class?

Formaldehyde may be terrific for preserving dead bodies and lab specimens, but it's not so great for the living. It can trigger health problems in almost every part of the body, and that goes for pets, too. Eyes, throat, skin, respiratory system, digestion, balance, all can be harmed just by inhaling a small amount of the stuff. Ingesting it can kill you.

A recent third problem with household products is the craze for *"antibacterial"* cleaners. These contain biocides which, in essence, are poisons (bio=life, cide=killer) not something you want on your skin, since whatever goes on your skin is absorbed into your body and transported to all your organs. The best defense against bacteria on your skin is a strong immune system and regular washing with soap and water, not a load of toxic chemicals.

If your cleaners contain detergent, scent and other problem substances, the best thing to do is put them into a box and take them to the *toxic waste dump.* In fact, no chemical-based cleaning product should *ever* be disposed of in the regular garbage! Regular garbage goes to a dump where the old products leak out of their containers into the soil and eventually into the water system for you to drink.

How can you tell if your cleaners are dangerous to your health? Look at the label for skull and crossbones, the word "corrosive", or any information about how health-friendly they are. Health-friendly? Most cleaners available in grocery stores are chemical-based and provide very little information about their contents, except the name of the extremely dangerous ingredient the emergency room doctor will need to know. In contrast, the more health-friendly cleaners tend to list all their ingredients, are biodegradable, free of artificial colors, and unscented or scented with plant-source materials, not chemicals.

Check your kitchen, bathroom, basement, and anywhere else you might have chemical cleaning products and get them out of your house! Even when they're sitting around in your closets they turn your home into a toxic swamp. Since their boxes, bottles, and spray cans are not completely sealed, these products continually outgas ammonia, chlorine, fragrance, ethanol, formaldehyde, petrochemicals, phenol, and other synthetics into your home air.

Even worse are the toxic fumes they send right into your face while you're using them. This may be a large part of the reason the homemakers mentioned earlier had such high cancer rates. They lived all day in the same house as the chemical products *and* they received direct exposure whenever they used those products, unlike other household members who would have had only secondary exposure. The long-term health effects of chemical household cleaners are obviously dangerous!

If you're one of those people who has always hated house-cleaning, the work itself may not be the problem. You may have used health-threatening products on a cleaning job and felt irritated, exhausted or depressed afterwards. Most likely you were reacting to the neurotoxic effects of the chemicals and your body was warning you to stay away from them. So don't let your cleaners steal your health! Collect them and ship them out. It's time to look at some safe products.

34. DISH WASHING.

Health-safe dish soap is particularly important. When you hand-wash dishes, you stand with your head above a sink full of hot water. Heat rises, so molecules of whatever product you put into the water fly straight up to your eyes, nose, and mouth where you inhale and ingest them. Even if you wear rubber gloves to protect your skin from absorbing the chemicals, any product that is in your sink also goes into *you*!

The majority of commercial dish-washing products are detergents. Detergent itself is a harmful chemical and so are the fragrance, alchohol, and dyes it contains. A better choice of product is one that contains no petrochemical derivatives, no colors or dyes, and is unscented or scented by plant materials rather than synthetics. This type of dish liquid tends to be biodegradable and may be available in your local grocery store, as more and more safe products are, or at a natural foods or environmental products store.

Two dish products we like and use are made by Nature Clean and Ecover. Both are liquid concentrates, so even though they may seem more expensive than regular dish detergent, you actually need less of them. They do not foam as heavily as dish detergents because they contain no foaming agents, but they are still cleaning your dishes. The Soap Factory makes a good grease-cutting biodegradable dish liquid.

For cutting grease and scrubbing pots or pans with cooked-on debris, nothing beats baking soda. Just sprinkle it on the area that needs cleaning and scrub. You can add baking soda, vinegar, or lemon juice to your dish water for extra grease-cutting power.

Baking soda will wash animal fat or chicken grease from your hands. First use a little soap on your skin, then sprinkle some baking soda into your sudsy hands and rub it around before rinsing. For convenience, keep a shaker jar or an open dish of baking soda with a small spoon in it near the sink for use on hands or dishes.

Dishwasher detergent is probably the single most difficult household product to replace. Ecover makes a good one. Another option is to buy a box of low-scent detergent from the grocery store. To reduce the amount of chlorine released into your home air, especially if any family member has breathing problems, look for a brand that uses enzymes instead of chlorine, such as Electrosol. Mix it with a box of unscented eco-friendly dishwasher powder, such as Nature Clean's, and store the mixture in a container with a lid to prevent outgassing. This way, you will have the cleaning power of detergent while using a product that is at least *half* safe and putting less detergent and chlorine down the drain. It's not the best solution, but it will at least reduce the amount of fragrance and chemical in your home and lessen your exposure to toxins.

Try to run your dishwasher when everyone is out of the house or well away from the kitchen. If possible, open a window to allow any scent or detergent fumes escaping from the dishwasher to leave your home. Debra Lynn Dadd recommends using sodium hexametaphosphate as a replacement for dishwasher detergent. It inhibits scale, cuts grease, and will clean your dishwasher as well as your dishes. To locate it, you may have to call your local allergy association.

Avoid antibacterial products. Salmonella bacteria can be killed by the high-temperature water from your hot water tap. Rather than risk your long-term health to antibacterial solutions, run the hot water until it steams to rinse cutting boards, utensils, and dishes you wash by hand. Most dishwashers have a sanitizing temperature feature which performs the same function. Another way to avoid bacteria is to use wooden cutting boards, not plastic ones.

Remember, even antibacterial products are not 100% effective and, because they contain biocides, they have the potential to overload your immune system. A strong, healthy immune system coupled with good hygiene habits is your best defense against ordinary bacteria. The so-called "superbugs" make a strong immune system even more important for every member of your family.

35. HOUSEHOLD CLEANERS.

Four safe products will clean your house: baking soda, borax, white vinegar and a biodegradable all-purpose cleaner or liquid natural soap. The bill for these cleaning products is incredibly low, and they won't cause health problems.

Yes, they actually work. These products don't have the powerful scents you may associate with cleaning and occasionally you may need to use a little more elbow grease, but there's a big plus side! Safe products are not strong enough to kill an adult with a few drops and they won't mutate your cells or cause cancer through long-term use.

Baking soda can be used to clean countertops, sinks, fridges and stoves inside and out, tile floors, and bathtubs. It's a terrific replacement for scrubbing powders. Use it straight, or add a little liquid soap. Stains on countertops will come out with baking soda. For tough stains, make a paste with baking soda and water and let it sit on the stain for several minutes—the longer, the better—before washing off.

Because baking soda deodorizes, you can wash food smells from wooden cutting boards or other surfaces with it. Use baking soda on your carpet to deodorize before vacuuming, instead of a chemical carpet product. Leave on for 10-15 minutes or longer and be sure the carpet is dry or the baking soda will stick and harden. (If this ever happens, it can be sponged out with plain water.)

Baking soda helps to keep your drain clean too. Pour a few spoonfuls down, followed by a half cup of vinegar, and put the plug in the drain. The baking soda and vinegar will fizz and bubble. Leave them for several minutes, then run very hot or boiling water down the drain. Serious clogs can be prevented by using a food trap, a little screen that fits into the drain opening—available from hardware or kitchen stores. Commercial drain cleaning products are one of the most dangerous items on the market. They *will* kill or damage you beyond repair if you happen to swallow them. Baking soda, on the other hand, is a *food* ingredient! Unlike other drain cleaners, it sends out no toxic fumes to poison your body.

Borax is a mineral so it is natural, however, it is *not* a food ingredient and should be handled with more care than baking soda. It has no fumes and contains no chemicals to build up in your system, so it is quite safe in that respect. But it is sometimes irritating to the skin, so don't spend a long time in contact with it, and definitely do not get it in your mouth or eyes. It can be used to disinfect. Use baking soda for cleaning in the kitchen, and borax for cleaning the bathroom or other areas where there is no food preparation going on.

Borax is great for sprinkling on a damp sponge to wash tiles, tubs, or shower stalls. Use it on stains. Be sure to rinse off with plain water. Pour some into the toilet instead of a toxic toilet cleaner and let sit for up to half an hour before scrubbing with the toilet brush. Add a little liquid soap, if necessary.

Because borax disinfects, it works well on mold. If you worry that cleaning with soap and water is not enough, you can use borax in place of antibacterial household products. As mentioned in the dishwashing chapter, very hot water also kills salmonella bacteria. Buy borax in the grocery store, in the laundry product section. Environmental products stores sell it in bulk. Another disinfectant with antibacterial properties is accelerated hydrogen peroxide.

Vinegar has almost as many uses as baking soda. Mix it with water (two parts water to one part vinegar) and put it into a spray bottle to clean mirrors, windows, glass table tops, and any other glass surfaces. Unlike commercial glass cleaners, vinegar contains no harmful ammonia or aerosol propellants, and it's a fraction of the price. It's great inside the car to clean windshield, windows, and mirror. If you don't like the smell of vinegar, add a few drops of lemon juice to the vinegar-and-water mixture.

Vinegar can be mixed with olive oil to polish wood furniture or floors. Traditional furniture polish is made from beeswax. On a recent television program, experts from a famous auction house explained the care of fine furniture. In the experts' opinion, spray furniture products should *never* be used as the petrochemical ingredients are not good for the wood and form a coating on surfaces which they said actually attracts dust! Vinegar and water can be used when dusting furniture—this mixture helps the dust-cloth pick up dust and does not damage surfaces.

You can use the same mixture for cleaning carpets and shoes. A saleswoman in a quality shoe store recommended I use a solution of vinegar and water to clean my leather footwear instead of a commercial product. According to her, it's especially good for taking salt marks off winter boots and will not harm leather.

All purpose cleaner or natural liquid soap. Look for an all purpose cleaner that is biodegradable and unscented or scented from plant sources. Nature Clean makes a "cleaning lotion", Ecover has an all-purpose cleanser, and the Soap Factory offers AA5 Concentrate, a multi-purpose cleaner that will do the job. These are replacements for any all-purpose cleaner you are currently using and can be used on most surfaces. Mix them with baking soda or borax for added cleaning power when scrubbing sinks, tub or tiles.

Another excellent multi-purpose cleaner is Orange Apeel which is especially good for problem jobs such as removing grease marks, fingerprints on walls, skunk smell, or cleaning up pet messes. Orange Apeel's citrus scent occurs naturally from its orange peel base ingredient.

For more information, read:
Baking Soda Bonanza by Peter A. Ciullo, HarperPerennial, NY 1995. Baking soda ideas for household cleaning, personal care, and recipes.
Vim Vinegar by Melodie Moore, HarperPerennial, NY 1997. Vinegar uses for household, personal care, garden, pets, and recipes.

PLASTICS

36. CONTAIN YOUR PLASTIC BAGS.

Plastic bags are a major source of indoor air pollution. They are soft plastic, and the softer the plastic, the looser the molecules. The molecules are so loose in plastic bags and plastic wrap, they float out into the air where you breathe them in. This floating away of molecules is how plastic bags outgas.

Plastic is a petrochemical, so continually breathing in molecules of plastic is a bit like standing beside a gas pump and breathing its fumes twenty-four hours a day. Some plastics are suspected carcinogens and may be responsible for bronchial, digestive, skin, and bladder problems.

To prevent trouble, the first thing to do is to go through your house and collect *all* the plastic bags you have stored away in drawers and closets.

When you do this, you may be shocked by the number of plastic bags you discover! Check the kitchen and pantry for plastic shopping bags, garbage bags, and plastic wrap, closets for clothes hung in dry cleaning bags, and drawers and boxes for seasonal items like gloves, scarves, sweaters, shoes, and gifts stored away inside plastic bags. Plastic bags may be "protecting" everything in your house except the humans!

The next step is to keep only the bags you *absolutely* need, perhaps some large bags for garbage and some smaller ones for other uses. *Throw the rest out.* Be ruthless about this. Plastics and petrochemicals have been linked to breast cancer in women and sterility in men, among other health problems, so the less exposure to them, the better.

Now, to keep the plastic bags you need from outgassing into your home air, store your bags in metal canisters or industrial-size glass jars. Cookie tins will work, although they have limited storage space. Especially useful are the large tins available in stores around holiday time—usually they are sold as containers of popcorn or chips. They are big enough to hold a good supply of bags and tend to be nicely decorated as well. You might keep one for garbage bags, one for plastic shopping bags, and a large cookie tin for sandwich and small bags.

Kitchen supply stores sell industrial sized glass jars with tight-closing metal lids that work equally well to prevent outgassing. Cardboard boxes will not keep petrochemical molecules out of your environment, so if you buy a box of garbage or other bags, take them out of the box and put them into a tin or jar.

To cut back on the number of bags that come into your home, take your own reusable shopping bags, baskets, or boxes to the grocery store or when running errands. Try keeping several cotton shopping bags on hand in your car, or take along a couple of big straw baskets for food shopping. This will dramatically reduce the number of plastic bags in your house. Consider carrying small or single purchases home without a bag.

Once you clear your home environment of plastic bags and other outgassing chemicals, the air in your house will be much cleaner and fresher.

37. STORING FOOD WITHOUT PLASTIC.

We live in such a plastic-dominated culture, it's hard to believe there was ever a time when plastic bags, wrap, bottles, and containers didn't exist. Yet plastics came into the kitchen only after World War II. Before that, people stored food in glass, paper, wax, metal, leather, cloth, baskets, pottery, and china. I remember my grandmother wrapping picnic sandwiches in a clean, damp tea towel—a pre-plastic era method of food preservation. The sandwiches were always fresh, cool, and delicious when we ate them.

Plastic bags and plastic wrap outgas molecules of petrochemical not only into your home environment, but into the *food* they contain! So when you store food in plastic, you get to eat all the plastic molecules that outgas into your food. The same thing tends to happen with soft plastic food containers.

Containers for foods like yogurt or margarine are best disposed of in the recycling bin. Don't use them to store leftovers, especially hot or warm leftovers, because heating plastic makes it outgas even *more*—and if the food is hot, it will heat the plastic it touches enough for some outgassing to occur. Plastic wrap and containers should never be used in the microwave because they will cook molecules of plastic into your food. Instead, use a glass or china dish and cover the food with a plate or paper towel.

Store food in glass jars. Glass jars can even go into the freezer. Leave a bit of air space between the food or liquid and the top of the jar so there's room for expansion. Glass usually freezes without any problems—just don't drop the jar on the floor when you take it out of the freezer. With liquids, I leave lots of air space and freeze the jars on their sides to prevent cracking. Once frozen, they can go upright.

Glass oven dishes with lids (Corning, Pyrex, etc.) work well to refrigerate larger items—leftover chicken, meat, casseroles. Put a piece of waxed paper or baking paper over the top of the food before putting the lid on, to keep out more air. This will not give you the same "seal" as plastic wrap, but it will keep foods in the fridge for three or four days. You can also buy elasticized food storage covers by mail from Gaiam products. Or just put leftovers in bowl with a plate over the top. Another storage option for larger items is a stainless steel bowl fitted with a plastic cover. Because only the cover is plastic, your food will not be touching it. These bowls range in size and are available where you buy kitchen wares.

Sometimes there is no fast, convenient way to store items like sandwiches, fresh meat, cheese or baked goods without using plastic bags. Wrap food items in waxed paper or baking paper before placing in plastic bags. That way they will be protected from touching the plastic and absorbing molecules of petrochemical. Be sure the items are not hot when you wrap and store them.

Vegetables can be stored without plastic in the crisper drawer with a damp tea towel laid over them. Remember to check the towel regularly to see if it needs re-dampening. Or look for cloth vegetable storage bags in natural foods and environmental products stores. You can also use 100% cotton pillowcases. Some vegetables, like broccoli and parsley, can be stored upright in a bowl or glass of water in the fridge, as if they were cut flowers. Store apples and pears away from other items as their skin releases a gas that will quick-ripen everything else. Put them in another drawer, in a covered bowl, or keep them out of the fridge altogether.

Plastic bags are not recyclable in our area so I try to keep my plastic garbage to a minimum by washing out bags and re-using them continually. Reusing bags is also a good idea because older plastic bags have already done some outgassing, so are slightly less volatile than new ones. Although plastic is convenient, it's best to use as little as possible around food. Plastics and petrochemicals may act as *xeno-estrogens* which are linked to cancer. As Andrew Weil, M.D., points out, xeno-estrogens are a possible reason for skyrocketing rates of breast cancer in industrialized nations (although men are probably no safer around plastics than women.) Since cancer is a disease that often takes years to develop, the fewer xeno-estrogens you encounter over your lifespan, the better your chances of maintaining good health.

In *Clinical Ecology*, Joseph and Alta Morgan recommend purchasing rolls of heavy sheet cellophane and cellophane bags to substitute for plastic wrap and bags. Cellophane is made from cellulose which is a plant-source material.

38. STORING CLOTHES AND OTHER ITEMS WITHOUT PLASTIC.

No house will be completely plastic-free. After all, pens, eyeglasses, computers, telephones, and t.v. remotes are made of plastic. Fortunately, these items are *hard* plastic, which does very little outgassing unless you set fire to it. (Never burn *any* plastic unless you want a lungful of deadly toxins.) You can tell hard plastics at a glance—they snap when you try to bend them, or crack if you smash them against a hard surface. Soft plastics, on the other hand, tend to bounce, bend easily, or scrunch.

Personal care and household products mostly come in plastic containers. Some highly chemical-sensitive people buy beautiful glass jars and bottles and transfer their products into them. This is a great idea but may not work for you. If not, leave your dish soap and shampoo in their plastic bottles and don't worry about it. The idea is not to be perfect, but to reduce your exposure to petrochemical molecules as much as possible.

A simple way to do this is to make sure you don't use plastic bags anywhere in your house to store clothing or other items. Instead of dry cleaning bags, cover hanging clothes with a dust sheet. Old tablecloths, sheets or any large piece of lightweight cotton fabric will do. Simply drape the cloth over the whole rack of clothing and tuck it around the clothes at each end so they are enclosed in a protective "tent". This works well to keep dust off seasonal and party wear.

For special outfits, purchase cotton garment bags through clothing, coat or speciality stores, or by mail order from Gaiam. Or simply buy a length of lightweight cotton fabric, make a small hole in the center to put the hook of the hanger through, and let the fabric drape down over your outfit to protect it.

Seasonal shoes, sweaters, and foldable clothing items can be stored in cardboard storage boxes, cloth bags or old pillowcases. Stationery and home furnishings stores sell attractive storage boxes with lids. When you buy boots or shoes, save the cardboard box to store them in. Socks, ribbons, and smaller items can go into cookie tins or glass jars.

Glass jars and cookie tins are very useful to store all sorts of household items from basement to attic. Use them for nails, screws, safety pins, hair pins, costume jewelry, bars of soap, cotton swabs, crayons, tape, felt-tipped markers, and anything else, especially items that contain chemical ingredients or arrive at your house in a plastic package. To keep your indoor air fresh, throw out plastic bags and wrappings as soon as you bring your purchases home from the store.

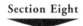

INDOOR AIR

39. SUPER-SEALED HOUSES.

New houses these days are so well sealed, they do a terrific job of keeping the indoor air confined. This enables you to control the temperature winter and summer—good news for your heating and air conditioning bills but not always for your health! In an airtight house, outgassing toxins stay indoors where they build up over time since they can't escape to the outdoors. Life in this toxic swamp can be very hard on you.

Older buildings have the advantage over newer ones, healthwise. They may not be as energy-efficient, but they typically have better air-exchange and ventilation, being less well-sealed. They also tend to have a lower proportion of synthetic building materials outgassing into the interior air, unless they have been extensively renovated. This is not to say everyone should look for an old house to live in, but that proper ventilation is absolutely necessary.

Air exchange means fresh air can flow in from the outdoors and stale air can flow out from the indoors. If you have a well-sealed house that does not have good air exchange, let some air in by opening a window. Even better, open two windows on opposite walls of the house so you get a good cross-draft.

Some people sleep with their bedroom windows open all year. Opening windows anywhere in the house, if only for a few minutes, is especially important in the winter. Winter is when your heating system goes on, potentially releasing molecules of fuel byproducts into your indoor air. Whatever toxins *are* in your home, heating and air conditioning systems help to circulate them throughout the entire house (which is why it's dangerous to keep outgassing toxic products indoors, even in the basement.) If you install an alarm system, try and get one that allows you to have windows open whenever you need to, day or night.

If opening windows doesn't work for you, an excellent solution to air exchange problems is to install a heat recovery ventilator—or HRV—system on your furnace. This device exchanges the air in the house, stale (chemically contaminated) for fresh, and ensures adequate ventilation. If you are sensitive to outdoor pollens and molds, you will need to insert an air filter into the system to clean the outdoor air prior to its circulation through your house. See Resource Guide for air cleaners and HRV's. When purchasing a household air filter system, check that the system is ducted to filter the house air, rather than only filtering the basement air.

Containing and eliminating toxins is especially important in a well-sealed house and will improve the effectiveness of any air filtration system. After you have removed the toxic substances from your home with help from the information in this book, open all the windows for several hours and give the place a good airing so any leftover fumes can blow away.

If you renovate, allow new materials enough time to outgas before you return to live in the rooms. Outgassing happens with all chemical products and materials containing them. For example, the smell of fresh paint is the paint outgassing—or releasing its chemical molecules—into your home air, where you inhale them. This also happens with chemically-treated fabrics and fibers for draperies and upholstery. Be careful around fresh paint, wallpaper, flooring, staining, refinishing, and other chemical processes. Even when the paint is low-odor and feels dry to the touch at the end of the job, molecules of it will still be in the air. Give chemicals and new materials lots of time to outgas, dry, and air out before you come near them.

One woman eliminated all her symptoms by changing her lifestyle habits. Then she painted her bedroom and immediately went back to sleeping in it. All her symptoms returned. She was in considerable distress until she moved out of the bedroom temporarily. She and her husband spent two weeks sleeping in another room while their bedroom outgassed and aired out, and eventually she returned to feeling well again.

One way to speed up the process and make renovations outgas quickly is with heat. Close all the windows, turn on the heat full blast and leave the house for several hours or a whole day. Pets should go, too. You may need to put plants outside or in winter, take them to a friend's temporarily. When you return, cover your nose and mouth, and open all the windows, allowing the fumes to blow away for an hour or so before you spend any time indoors.

Another way to keep the air in your house fresh is to use plants. Most leafy green plants will contribute to fresher air somewhat. But there are several varieties that are top performers at clearing chemical vapors and fumes from indoor air.

NASA and other research groups have tested different plants for their air-cleaning abilities by putting them in sealed rooms full of toxic fumes. (Poor plants!) Here are some of the plants they found most successfully removed chemical toxins such as formaldehyde from the air: English ivy, rubber plant, spider plant, areca palm, bamboo palm, aloe vera, boston fern, chrysanthemum, dendrobium orchid, peace lily, and Dracaena 'Janet Craig'. Ask for these at your local plant shop. If you want to know more about toxin-removing houseplants, read *How to Grow Fresh Air*, by B.C. Wolverton (Viking Penguin, 1996).

Wouldn't it be great if all you had to do to improve your health and indoor air was to buy a few plants? The drawback to these marvels of nature is that when you water their soil it releases mold into the air. If you have symptoms relating to mold sensitivity, you will be better off without indoor plants, no matter how much you love them. Whether the toxins are natural or synthetic, the less direct and indirect toxic exposure you receive, the healthier you and your descendants will be. Avoidance of toxins is always the first line of defence.

40. THE TROUBLE WITH MOLD.

Mold is very important—if it weren't for molds, organic materials would never break down and return to the soil from whence they came. Yet, despite mold's beneficial aspects, it can be irritating to humans.

Do you feel melancholy and tired after a rainfall, or cough when you walk through fallen leaves? If so, you've been affected by mold. Marshall Mandell, M.D., connects mold with asthma and breathing problems. Doris Rapp, M.D., associates it with depression, frequent need to urinate, and chronic tiredness. According to A.V. Constantini, M.D., director of the WHO Collaborating Center for Mycotoxins in Food, molds and fungus (mycotoxins) are powerful contributing factors in many disease conditions, including athlerosclerosis, obesity, asthma, arthritis, cancer, gout, and hyperactivity.

There are thousands of molds in existence, travelling through the air, indoors and out. They like moisture, earth, and basements. Molds are in carpets, older mattresses, bathrooms, aquariums, cottages, furniture that is not kept in completely dry surroundings, camping equipment, gardens (earth is damp and always moldy), the soil of potted plants, fallen leaves, and the outdoors—mostly in spring or fall when there is moisture from melting snow or rainfall. There is less mold *during* the rain than after, as the falling rain tends to wash away mold, but once it stops, the mold from damp soil and rotting vegetation gets into the air again.

As with chemicals, the best approach to mold is avoidance. If you or your family members have any kind of breathing problem, beware of buying a house in a forest or beside a lake or swamp. Be sure your house has a very dry basement or, better yet, no basement. The mold factor is one reason asthmatics and people with allergies do well in locations like Arizona where the climate is dry. If you move to Arizona, take advantage of the mold-free desert landscape and don't put in a "moldy" lawn.

Inside your house, keep moldy or potentially moldy areas clean and dry. Run the fan in the bathroom when bathing or showering, don't have your bedroom in the basement, and use a dehumidifier when necessary. Mold is not something you can cover up with another smell. When it comes to mold, room deodorizers do nothing but add to your body's toxic load.

Two effective mold cleaners are borax in water, and hydrogen peroxide or accelerated hydrogen peroxide. Kill mold with heat from a blow dryer or portable heater, then wipe or vaccuum it up. If the mold is bad enough that you feel you have to use bleach on it, cover your nose and mouth, work as quickly as possible, and then keep the area dry or clean it regularly with borax or hydrogen peroxide so mold does not grow again. Bleach is a very dangerous chemical, so do everything you can to avoid using it.

Put houseplants outside or confine them to one small area of the house. People with asthma will do well to avoid houseplants and aquariums completely. If you have indoor plants, water them just before you go out, so the soil will dry a little before you return. That way, you won't have to spend time breathing in fresh, floating mold spores right from the wet soil. You can also try covering the soil surface with aquarium rocks to keep mold in the pot. If you love indoor plants and you have no breathing problems, the lower you keep your total toxic load from chemicals and other sources, the less you will be stressed by mold from the plants.

Broadloom is a primary source of mold, growing a potential 10 million micro-organisms per square foot! Sprinkle broadloom regularly with borax to discourage mold growth, then vacuum. Better yet, remove broadloom completely and have sealed wood or ceramic tile floors, particularly in the bedroom.

It is impossible to avoid all molds, but you can give your immune system a tremendous boost in resisting the negative effects of mold and fungus by keeping them to a minimum in your home and food. (for information about mold and fungus in diet, see chapter on *moldy and yeasty foods.*)

41. ABOUT SCENT.

Scented products are a primary source of indoor air pollution. Before the twentieth century, scents came from natural sources: flowers, plants, and scent glands from animals. The fixatives used to hold the scent and keep it from disappearing were vegetable or animal oils. Because these materials were expensive—it could take pounds of flower petals just to make an ounce or two of fragrance—and sometimes difficult to obtain, many who could afford perfume were wealthy and titled. In general, most people did not receive a lot of scent exposure.

Today, the chemical industry synthesizes scents and "fixes" them with chemicals such as formaldehyde. Formaldehyde is a suspected carcinogen and, like scent, can act as a neurotoxin, throwing off the way you think, feel and behave. Headaches, dizziness, fuzzy thinking, tiredness, temper tantrums, and mood swings are possible outcomes. If you spend a lot of time driving, doing precision mental or physical work, using knives or other sharp tools or relying on your people skills, anything containing formaldehyde is *not* your best friend.

Synthetic fragrance has made scent much less expensive to produce and, as a result, *everything* we use can be perfumed. In North America, so many products are pefumed, going unscented seems unusual! There's an irony to this. Perfumers developed their art, particularly in Europe, not just because humans like fragrance but to cover up the less appealing odors inevitable in crowded cities where humans, horses, donkeys and other creatures shared streets and sometimes houses, and sanitation was limited or non-existent for hundreds of years.

In this day and age, we have bathing and sanitary facilities unparalleled since the fall of Rome. We are cleaner than Western humans have been for upwards of 2,000 years. Our clothes are cleaner and easier to keep clean and our streets and houses are free of droppings from humans and beasts of burden. Given these superior conditions, while perfume may be nice, it is hardly *necessary*.

By perfume, I don't mean just the expensive designer liquid in the fancy bottle from Paris. I mean fragrance in every household or personal care product, from dish and laundry detergent to deodorant. When you look around your house, you may be as surprised as I was to discover how many products contain scent! They include laundry, dish, and household cleaning products, scented hangers, candles, sachets, pillows, and stationery, some socks, some art supplies, especially those for children, some toy items, air fresheners, incense, pot pourri, towelettes, wipes, powders, and all personal care products.

One way to tell if scented products seem to agree with you or if you are poisoning yourself unknowingly is to go off *all* scented products for a week Going off them means collecting all the scented products in your house and putting them in a garage or other place where they cannot affect your indoor air, breathing, and skin. You will need to have some unscented replacement products on hand. At the end of the scent-free week, try the products again. If you have *any* type of reaction: headache, digestive trouble, skin problem, runny eyes or nose, food cravings, depression, anxiety, rage, weepiness, (check back to your list in chapter 3) not just immediately but over the next few days, you are probably better off not to use these products.

If you experience no reaction at all, you may be one of those rare people whose immune system is strong enough to deal with the daily onslaught of chemical. For the present. However, you may want to consider the long-terms effects of accumulating toxins in your body, especially if you plan to have children (this applies to both women and men). Many of the ingredients in fragrance are not listed on packages and are highly toxic, particularly after they have collected in your cells for a few years. The safest choice is to move directly to unscented products for all purposes.

42. KEEP PAINT, GLUE, AND SOLVENTS OUT OF YOUR INDOOR AIR.

To track down additional sources of indoor pollution, look through your basement or other storage area or workroom for toxic products you seldom use. Are you storing odds and ends of old paint from redecorating, dried-out sealers and glues, solvents, and rusting squirt cans of oil? If so, collect this medley of outgassing toxins in a box and take it to the toxic waste dump.

These liquid chemicals are volatile, from the Latin *volare* which means "to fly". Molecules of volatile chemicals are always ready to fly out, or outgas, into your air.

As soon as you open a can of liquid chemicals like paint or solvent, the fumes fly out. If you can smell them, you're bringing them into your body.

But even after you no longer smell the chemicals, they continue outgassing, probably because it's impossible to reseal an opened container as tightly as it was first sealed in the factory. Ever notice how old cans of paint or glue tend to dry out, even when you've put the lid back on? The stuff is drying right into the air you breathe. Cans of products like oil may have outgassing drips or spills along the sides, once used. Then there are spray chemical products—paints, oils—that should never be used inside your home. Spraying a chemical makes it outgas at lightspeed.

In *Nontoxic, Natural, and Earthwise*, Debra Lynn Dadd mentions a Johns Hopkins Hospital study in which paints were found to contain a possible 300 toxic chemicals and 150 carcinogens. So, if you want to reduce your total toxic load and breathe health-supporting indoor air, keep powerful chemicals out of your home!

You might wonder why it's okay to store tins of plastic bags in your home but not paint and other chemicals that *arrive* in a can. Plastic bags and other soft plastics may have loose molecules, but, unlike more volatile chemicals, once they're in the can, they stay there (until you open it, but you still have less outgassing this way than if the bags are lying all over your house.)

If you use volatile chemical products, store them in the garage or shed or a place not connected with your indoor air circulation. When working with toxic products, wear a mask over your nose and mouth to avoid inhaling them, and be sure you use them only in well-ventilated areas. You will want to protect yourself especially around any product that has the skull and crossbones on the label.

Companies who manufacture these products use this symbol to tell you you are working with hazardous chemicals that will seriously damage your health if you're not careful. Sometimes the label warns you not to swallow the product, but even the fumes can cause severe long-term health problems as well as neurotoxic mood- and behavior-altering effects including memory loss, outbursts of rage or violent behavior, loss of motor control, and deadening of sense of smell.

Never dump these products down the sink. They end up in your water system and municipal filtration does not filter chemicals out. (Rule of thumb for all products: if you pour it down the sink today, you drink it tomorrow.) The easiest way to dispose of toxic products is at the toxic waste facility—in our city, they even accept the water used to wash paint out of paintbrushes. For the sake of your health, you may decide you want to buy safer alternatives to these products from environmental products suppliers, such as Grassroots, Healthy Home Services, Gaiam or Greenhome (see Resources).

43. NATURAL GAS.

If you've cooked with gas, you know gas burners give you full heat instantly and allow rapid changes of temperature that aren't possible with electric stoves. But is it safe?

I love cooking with gas, so I'm sorry to say there are some major health concerns with this fuel. Gas stoves and furnaces, particularly older models, can release molecules of carbon monoxide and nitrogen dioxide into your home environment. Nitrogen dioxide is a carcinogen precursor. It damages the mucous membranes of the lungs, so it is very dangerous for asthmatics. *If there is an asthmatic in your household, do not buy gas appliances!* Use an electric stove, and some other form of heating than forced air gas heat. Do not run gas lines through your basement to reach outdoor barbecues or pool heaters.

Even if you're not asthmatic, it's wise to be very careful around natural gas. Nitrogen dioxide interferes with the way oxygen is transported in your body, and it affects the brain negatively, resulting in memory loss, fatigue, confusion, depression, and apathy. Long-term exposure will cause damage to brain structure and functioning. Circulatory problems are also a possibility. The stress of natural gas toxins on the immune system make trouble for the body's abililty to heal infections.

Newer gas stoves with electronic pilot lights and high-efficiency furnaces do not leak gas fumes as much as do older models. However, recent studies show that *even in very tiny amounts*, these chemical fumes can cause physical damage. If you have gas appliances, be sure your house is well-ventilated. *Install a fume hood that vents to the outdoors* over your stove and use it every time you ignite the burners or oven. At the very least, open a window when you fire up your stove, so the gas fumes that are released can flow outside. The fewer toxic molecules your body has to deal with, the better you will operate on all levels—mentally, physically, and emotionally.

44. SOURCES OF CHEMICAL YOU MIGHT NEVER SUSPECT.

Do you have paraffin candles, oil-burning lamps, tape, art supplies, new books, magazines, newspapers, and gift wrap in your home or office? These items are outgassing chemicals into your indoor environment and sneakily eroding your health. Still, you might need some of them occasionally. The plan, in this case, is to use and store these items so your exposure to any toxins is minimized.

Most candles are paraffin, a petrochemical product. If you've cleared your house of scents and chemicals, using a few candles now and then probably won't cause you too much damage, unless your immune system is already compromised (if you're sick or have a chronic condition). Just follow these simple steps: Avoid breathing in smoke, air out the room after burning candles, and when not in use store new and partly-used candles in cookie tins or large jars to seal their chemicals away from your indoor air.

When your indoor air is clean and mostly chemical-free, you may notice your eyes water and hurt when you burn paraffin candles. Natural-source candles are unlikely to cause such reactions. These include beeswax and bayberry (the real thing, not just the scent) as well as corn-based and soybean oil-based candles. Your local natural food or environmental products store will carry non-toxic candles.

Paraffin and other oil lamps release petrochemical fumes when you burn them, and outgas chemical molecules when they're sitting around waiting to be used. Oil lamps have been compared to Molotov cocktails since they are incendiary fuel with a wick. Scary! If you have these lamps primarily for decoration, leave the oil out of them.

Newspapers, magazines, and books are printed with petrochemically-based inks or soy-based inks that may contain some petrochemical derivatives. Either way, you might experience dizzyness, nausea, exhaustion, dyslexia, or sudden behavior changes when confronted with the odor of a freshly printed product. You could even react like one man who found he wanted to go back to sleep after reading the newspaper over breakfast!

To avoid toxic results, open up that newspaper or book in a porch or garage and leave it to outgas for several hours or days before bringing it indoors to read. Even a few minutes of ruffling the pages outdoors can make a difference—try not to stand with your face right over the pages. Sunlight speeds the outgassing process, as does heat.

Or open a new book, ruffle the pages, and set it upright before a heater or vent indoors for several hours or days before reading. The point is that you want to get the chemical smell out before you spend time with the reading material in front of your face, where the ink fumes will waft directly into your eyes, nose, and mouth.

Whatever you do, *don't* store a pile of brand-new books and magazines right next to your bed. This stresses your system and makes it hard for you to wake up feeling rested. You need fresh air when you sleep, not a pile of chemicals next to your head where you breathe them in all night. In fact, it's probably best to shelve your books and mags in a room other than your bedroom. Just bring in one or two to read, and put them in a drawer or somewhere away from your head when you go to sleep.

Library books and newspapers are great because, after they've been read by three or four people, all the pages have been opened and done their outgassing. I love new books, but once I learned about toxic inks, my buying habits changed significantly. I used to look for the freshest and least handled copy in the bookstore. Now I take the one that looks like it has been opened a few times.

Gift wrapping paper is another source of chemical-based inks. These papers are heavily coated with colors and finishes which outgas toxic fumes. If you burn them in your fireplace, the fumes are even worse (like burning plastic). In general, the more colorful and glossy the wrapping paper, the more toxic it is likely to be.

Try creative alternatives to toxic wrapping paper. Use cloth bags or fabric wrapping for gifts, or save paper gift bags that have had some time to outgas, and reuse them. Inexpensive tea towels decorated with holiday themes are another option. Or buy rolls of plain brown paper from the stationery or office supply store. You, your children, and your inner child can write, draw or paint on this type of wrapping or decorate it with colorful ribbons. Brown paper is low in chemical toxicity, so can be burned in the fireplace.

Use art supplies, glue, tape, art paints, felt-tipped markers, and brush cleaners where there is good ventilation, near an open window, an air filter machine or outdoors. When you use them professionally, consider installing a fume hood or air exchanger to bring in lots of fresh air. Store art materials in large tins and/or jars with tight-fitting lids to prevent them outgassing into your home air.

45. FRESHENING INDOOR AIR.

In our city, chemical air fresheners are considered so toxic, they must be disposed of at the local toxic waste facility! These products often work by masking other odors with a strong scent, or by deactivating your full ability to smell.

Room sprays are a fast, effective way to coat the inside of your entire home, not to mention your lungs, with toxins. I once had a part time job in a flower shop which sold a pricey chemical-based spray air "freshener". The great thing about it was, when the glue from price tags got stuck on ornaments or china pots, we simply used a little of this room spray on it. The spray dissolved the glue in no time, enabling us to wipe it off easily. That was back in the days before I figured out that if room spray was dissolving hardened glue, it probably wasn't all that good for *me*, either. Even a product as innocent-looking as pot pourri outgasses toxic chemicals into your home, unless it is made with plant-source essential oils only.

Here are some safer ways to deodorize your house:

Baking soda tops the list of deodorizers. Unlike room deodorants that only cover up the odors, it actually *absorbs* them. Sprinkle it on your carpets, and leave it there for 15 to 30 minutes before vacuuming. Put an open dish of it in your refrigerator and another near the stove. If you have a fire on the stove, you can dump it on the flames to put them out. Cooking odors are best eliminated with a fan, particularly if you vent your fume hood to the outdoors.

Dishes of baking soda can be placed in any odorous area of your house—although, once the toxins are cleared from your home, you are unlikely to have bad smells except occasionally in the kitchen or bathroom. Since baking soda is edible, it will not harm pets if they happen to lick it. Sprinkle it into your kitchen garbage can before putting in the plastic bag liner. Dust kitty litter with baking soda to keep the smell down. It will not harm your cat if she gets it on her feet.

If your house smells because your pet has just had an accident on the carpet, clean the spot with Orange Apeel. This citrus-based solution will scent your air naturally while it cleans.

Another technique for keeping bad smells out of your house is to separate your kitchen garbage. This means putting food garbage into a separate container from the rest of your garbage. Food waste tends to smell worst because it is decomposing. In my house, food garbage goes into an enamel bucket with a lid, purchased at a kitchen supply store. When this is full, it is emptied into the composter in the back yard. That takes care of all the vegetable and fruit waste. Meat waste—bones, fat, and so forth—goes into a container in the fridge and is thrown into the kitchen garbage bag on garbage collection day. This keeps it from spending several days rotting in the kitchen garbage can. If you have a shed or garage adjoining your house, you can keep a garbage receptacle for meat waste there. To further keep down smells in your kitchen garbage, rinse meat papers and messy plastic food bags before throwing them out.

In the bathroom, if someone has left a bad smell behind them, light a match in the room and let it burn for a couple of seconds. The smell "burns up". Lighting a candle in the bathroom can have a similar effect.

Perhaps your interest in air fresheners is to make your house smell nice, rather than to cover up unpleasant odors. You don't have to use chemicals to scent your house. There are other ways, safer for your health.

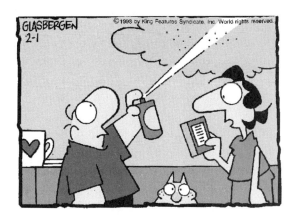

"Guaranteed to cover up cooking odors, pet odors and odors caused by the decay of civilized society."

To make your house smell delicious, simmer a pot of apple cider, cloves, and cinnamon on the stove. Even a small amount mixed with water (to make it last longer) and heated will fill your house with a wonderful scent, without giving you a dose of formaldehyde or other toxins. This spiced apple scent is particularly appealing for autumn and winter celebrations. Simmer water with a spoonful of herbs—rosemary has a wonderful fragrance—or slices of orange and lemon for a citrus scent or a few drops of vanilla extract. In earlier times, people sprinkled lavender in their clothing drawers against moths. If you've had a balsam Christmas tree or walked in a grove of balsam trees, you know how well they scent the air. Save a bowl of needles from your Christmas tree.

For general air clearing, plants do a wonderful job if you tolerate the mold in their soil. Even without plants, once you eliminate toxins and artificial scents from your interiors, you will find your sense of smell improves and you will love the cleaner air quality in your home!

INTERIORS, FURNISHINGS & RENOVATIONS

46. HOW TO HAVE A HEALTHY FLOOR.

Carpeting, especially new broadloom fresh from the factory, is *full* of outgassing petrochemicals, formaldehyde, pesticides, and other chemicals including neurotoxins and carcinogens. Unless your carpets are 100% cotton, wool, or silk (and sometimes even when they are), you are better off without them. New houses typically contain broadloom and are so well sealed and insulated, the chemicals stay right in the house creating a toxic environment that can literally make you sick.

The bedroom is *the* most important room to make into a health-supporting environment. If you can't bear to rip out all your broadloom, at least remove it from your bedrooms. That way, you won't have to inhale carpet toxins all night while you're trying to rest and recuperate. If you've stored scraps or ends of carpet in closets or basement, put them in the garage or throw them out.

Broadloom that is five or more years old has usually outgassed most of its chemicals. But at this point other problems take precedence. Since older carpets are impossible to clean thoroughly, even by professionals, they breed dust-mites, molds, and fungus, all of which cause health problems. One study discovered ten million micro-organisms per square foot growing in carpets!

The two healthiest floor surfaces are hardwood, sealed with low-emission wood sealer, and ceramic tile. Laminate wood flooring and cork flooring are also good choices. These four flooring options are easy to clean, non-allergenic, and do not collect dust and organic growths permanently the way carpets do. When you change your flooring from carpeting to one of these four you'll be astounded at how much cleaner your home looks and feels.

When you remove broadloom, you may find the floor beneath is plywood. If you live in a recently-built house, you may also have an unexpected cleaning job to do, like one friend of ours. When she lifted the broadloom, she found lots of sawdust and other messy remnants that had simply been left under the carpet by the builders! Both plywood and particle board contain formaldehyde that must be prevented from outgassing. This outgassing goes right through broadloom, which is porous and will not shield you from the formaldehyde in the flooring. If you're not ready to install a health-safe flooring surface for some time after you lift the broadloom, seal the plywood or particle board with wood sealer. Floors can also be painted before sealing to look like carpets with borders and other creative touches or finished simply with elegant solid colors. Crystal Shield is a wood sealer that seals in formaldehyde.

If you live where winters are cold and snowy, you may worry that a ceramic tile floor will be too cold. Tile *is* a cooler material than wood but if you wear shoes or slippers in the winter, floor surface makes no difference unless you're planning to sit on it. The Romans used to heat their tile floors by piping hot air beneath them. For today's equivalent, look for radiant floor heating, the contemporary way to heat ceramic tile floors.

Another factor that will affect the apparent warmth of your ceramic tile floor is color. Large terra cotta-colored tiles that look as if they have the glow of the Tuscan sun baked into them appear much warmer than small sterile white tiles.

With tile or hardwood, when your child needs a padded surface to play on, try layering two or three cotton thermal blankets on the floor. (These can go into the washing machine and dryer). Or give your children big cushions, pillows or cork pads to sit on. Washable sheepskins or lambskins for children who are not wool-sensitive are another good choice.

There may be an area in your house where you feel you absolutely must have carpet. This might be the spot where you step out of bed, the bathroom floor beside the tub, or the place where the dog or cat loves to curl up. Use a small cotton rug you can throw into the washer and dryer on a regular basis. Check to make sure there is no petrochemical (plasticized or rubbery) backing on these carpets. It's a good idea to wash them as soon as you bring them home, before your feet, pets, or children come in contact with them, to remove any pesticides or preservative-type chemicals that are in some cotton products.

When you want something larger than a throw rug, cotton or low-pile wool area rugs are a good choice. One of the beauties of wool is its natural ability to resist flame, so it is a good choice for in front of a fireplace. Be sure the carpet you choose has no petrochemical backing and has *not* been moth-proofed or fire-proofed. Rather than shampooing the carpet which wets the carpet and may result in mold growth, put it outside in the blazing summer sun for several hours at least once a year to kill any dust-mites or other organic growths and shake, beat, or sweep it while outdoors.

47. HEALTHY FABRICS FOR INTERIORS.

Choosing fabric? Think natural-source as opposed to synthetic. Man-made fibers are synthesized from petrochemicals. Additional chemicals make them water- and stain-repellent, fireproof, wrinkle-free, and easy-care. Such fabrics may seem easy to look after but their effects on your health are not.

Formaldehyde features in the production of synthetic fabrics and poly-cotton blends. The chemicals in new curtains and upholstery outgas into your indoor air, adding toxins to your home environment. Your clothing is not a barrier to chemical effects when you sit on upholstery.

Fabric dyes are a problem for some people, especially in the darker color ranges. Most dyes are from a petrochemical source and may contain heavy metals, so if you have a young child who puts everything into his or her mouth, be careful with heavily dyed fabrics. *Very* sensitive people can react to dyes simply by touching the fabric. With any fabric that's not 100% colorfast, molecules of the dye can leak into your skin just as it does into water.

When purchasing curtain and upholstery fabrics or upholstered furniture, here are some factors to consider. In general, the less treated, finished, and dyed a fabric is, the better. Be wary of fabrics that contain water- and stain-repellents, or manufacturers who offer to apply a stain-repellent coating. Instead of chemical stain-resistant coatings on your upholstery, consider removable covers in natural-fiber fabrics that can be washed with water (not dry cleaned). Avoid poly-cotton blends. If there are babies and small children or people with chronic health conditions in your family, look for light-colored or natural, undyed fabrics. Wool upholstery fabric, like wool carpets, should *not* be moth-proofed.

Natural fibers include cotton, wool, linen, ramie, flax, hemp, and silk. Any of these are excellent choices, particularly a washable cotton or hemp, or a cotton/silk or cotton/linen blend. Before using, wash the fabric in the washing machine with a non-toxic cleaner (see chapter on laundry products) to remove insecticides and other chemicals left over from the growing and manufacturing process. You can then have the fabric made into curtains or furniture covering. Be sure to tell the draper or upholsterer not to use any chemical treatments on your material. No stain repellents, moth- or fire-proofing.

The great thing about washable fabrics is you don't have to pay for dry cleaning or suffer through the outgassing of dangerous dry cleaning chemicals into your home air. If you have no option but to buy a treated or synthetic fabric because that's what happens to be on the furniture you want, let it outgas for several days if possible in a garage or space not connected with your indoor air, or put it outside in the hot sun for several hours to get rid of that "new" chemical smell.

When choosing shower curtains, tablecloths, placemats, seat covers, and plastic mats for wet boots, watch out for vinyl products. Products containing vinyl release vinyl chloride, a carcinogen and mutagen (mutagens affect your genes). Buy cotton or linen tablecloths, placemats, and seat covers. Or look for placemats in other natural materials like wood, straw or hemp, and floor mats in jute, cotton, cork or coconut fiber.

A plastic shower curtain can be replaced with a glass door or a cotton shower curtain. If you choose to keep your plastic shower curtain, be scrupulous about removing all other sources of vinyl and plastic to minimize your chemical exposure. When buying a new plastic shower curtain, be sure to open the package *outdoors*, unfold the curtain, and let it outgas for a couple of days before bringing it indoors. Hot sun speeds up the process. This will cut down on some of the worst exposure, as products always outgas most when they're new.

48. HEALTHY FURNITURE.

In a perfect world, furniture could all be made of solid wood. In the real world of diminishing wood sources, lots of new furniture is made with particleboard, particularly on the sides that don't show—the back, the bottom, underneath the drawers or inside veneered cupboard doors. Particleboard and plywood contain phenols, plastics, and formaldehyde, a suspected carcinogen and known irritant implicated in asthma, insomnia, and other reactions.

But you don't have to throw out your current furnishings even if they are made with these materials. To keep your particleboard furniture from causing you problems, seal it with several coats (at least three) of a low-emission wood sealer, such as Crystal Aire. Make sure to coat all surfaces. The veneer side must be sealed as well as the sides where you can actually see the particleboard, since veneer does not prevent formaldehyde from outgassing. The undersides of kitchen counters and cabinets may need sealing.

The most important room to keep free of particleboard furniture is an infant's or child's bedroom. According to Debra Lynn Dadd, there is evidence that formaldehyde may be related to Sudden Infant Death Syndrome.

Most retail baby cribs have particleboard supporting the mattress. Cribs and children's beds and other furniture can be sealed with Crystal Aire. Chemicals in bedding and furniture can be part of childhood bedwetting problems.

If you are buying solid wood furniture, examine all sides of the piece, including the drawers, if any, to be sure no one cheated and put in a little particleboard. Also keep in mind that some people are sensitive to wood resins (sap) present in solid wood furniture. If this becomes a problem, you can seal or paint the furniture. You might also consider furniture made of metal or metal and glass, wicker, and bamboo.

A final consideration for furniture is the filling in the upholstery cushions. Once upon a time, cushions and seats were stuffed with horsehair, straw, cotton, wool, feathers or kapok. These days, most padded furniture is stuffed with some form of petrochemical foam. Not everyone will need to change their couch to a completely natural one. If you're okay with a polyester-stuffed pillow on your bed, you'll be fine with this as furniture stuffing.

However, if you are extremely chemically-sensitive, you may wish to have a couch made over with a natural stuffing and covering. Wool batting free of moth-proofing or cotton batting that contains no petrochemicals or pesticides are good choices. The cleanest stuffing of all is probably silk batting. Be cautious about choosing feather or down stuffing. Apart from the cost of a down-filled couch, which could be prohibitive, many people do not tolerate feathers well.

49. RENOVATIONS AND DECORATING.

Want to renovate or decorate and stay healthy? Here are some ideas to keep in mind.

For almost every building or decorating product that's full of toxic chemicals, there are healthier alternatives on the market. Ask in the paint, wallpaper, and hardware stores about products that are environmentally friendly or designed for people with allergies, whether or not *you* have allergies. What you're looking for are products with the lowest levels of toxins—they will be more health-supporting than the usual version. You can also shop for them at environmental product stores, mail order outlets, and pharmacies that specialize in health products.

Paint and Wallpaper:

Most paint companies now offer low-odor latex that cleans up with water. Use these products with *lots* of ventilation—in other words, with your windows wide open. Wear a mask or scarf over your nose and mouth if you are doing the painting yourself. Be particularly careful if you have bowel, skin or breathing problems. 'Low-odor' is *not* the same as chemical-free. Instead of washing the paint from brushes and rollers down the sink, wash them in a container, then a) put the container, uncovered, in a garage or shed where no animals or children can get at it and let the water evaporate (once water is gone, the container can be thrown out), or b) pour the paint-laden wash water into a bottle with a tight lid, such as an empty water bottle, and take it to the toxic dump for disposal.

Summer is the best time to paint indoors or wallpaper because you can keep your windows open. If you are pollen-sensitive, don't paint with open windows during the height of pollen season. Your local weather station or allergy association can usually tell you when pollen is peaking. Fresh wallpaper inks and glues need to outgas just like paint. Painting in winter means keeping the windows shut and having paint fumes rotate through your house via the heating system. Allow at least a week for latex and wallpaper to outgas and *do not sleep in a freshly painted or wallpapered room* until it has outgassed for several days. Ideally, you would sleep in another house entirely. Oil paint or other oil finishes in your house can take a year to outgas!

Children and Pets:

Babies and children are much more susceptible to toxins than adults because their immune systems are still developing. They need to be protected from the chemicals in fresh paint and other building and decorating supplies, as do pets. Children whose bodies are struggling with chemical toxins may take extra time to recover from seasonal colds and viruses. When possible, send your kids to a friend or relative during painting or renovation work.

Keep pets, including fish and birds, in a safe, toxin-free place until the danger of chemical exposure to renovation materials is past. Unlike humans, pets will groom plaster dust, wet paint, glue, floor sealers, and other building materials from their feet and bodies with their mouths, so are in danger of direct internal and external exposure. Pets should not be allowed on building sites, where their unprotected paws may be punctured by splinters, loose nails, and sharp tools.

If you are preparing a room for a new baby, paint or wallpaper *well* in advance of the birth so the room has time to outgas before the baby moves in. Many cases of colicky, sleepless, and upset babies who are otherwise healthy may result from exposure to chemicals in new bedding, cribs made with particle board, recent decorating, fabric softener, and personal care products. For babies, the more natural, unscented, and chemical-free the product, the better. To avoid passing on toxins to the fetus, pregnant women should probably not paint rooms or furniture.

Insulation, Plywood and Particle-board:

Exercise great caution around renovations that involve insulation, raw plywood, and particleboard. Cover your nose and mouth when using these materials. As with furniture, seal plywood and particleboard with Crystal Aire or Crystal Shield. Fiberglass insulation may be contaminated with asbestos which is a carcinogen and harms the lungs. You can order fiberglass in paper or aluminum wrapped bats so you never touch the actual insulation. If you use unwrapped fiberglass, cover as much of your skin, hair, nose, and mouth as possible to avoid contacting or breathing in fibers. A better choice would be cellulose insulation or mineral wool insulation.

Block off the area being renovated from the rest of the house so that chemicals, sawdust, particles of insulation, and other materials do not enter your living area. When you hire outside help, have them screen off the work area—even if this involves taping up a large sheet of plastic to seal off the area. Better a few molecules of plastic than a high dose of varied toxins and fresh chemical particles spread throughout your house. You could also use an old cotton sheet or a drop cloth.

Pressure-treated wood:

Pressure-treated wood is treated with *cyanide*. It is *exceptionally* dangerous. An untreated splinter can lead to amputation or fatality. *Splinters from pressure-treated wood are extremely serious. If you get one, go immediately to a hospital emergency, even if you have taken the splinter out.* You may need drug treatment to avoid poisoning.

Do not have decks, docks, garden benches or deck seats made of pressure-treated wood. Even if they are painted or stained, this is not a sufficient seal. As time goes on, and the stain wears down, you or your children or pets could get a splinter in bare feet or hands. A house and dock builder told me pressure-treated wood lasts no longer than regular wood for outdoor uses, so if you are considering it for longevity, you may as well go with untreated wood. An alternative to pressure-treated wood is to use Lifetime wood treatment—a natural wood preservative that, once applied, eliminates the need to paint or stain the wood. Available from Healthy Home Services. (see Resources.)

Toxic fume barrier:

If your garage is attached to your house or you are adding on a room above the garage, use a vapor barrier to keep gas, oil, and other toxic fumes out of your house. In *Poisoning Our Children*, Nancy Sokol Green recommends lining the adjoining garage wall or ceiling with Dennyfoil, stock #242 or #245, which is free of toxic chemical additives and provides protection against all types of chemical vapors.

For more information, read:
Healthy by Design-Building and Remodelling Solutions for Creating Healthy Homes, by David Rousseau and James Wasley, Hartley & Marks, Port Roberts, WA 1997.
The Natural House Catalog-Everything You Need to Know to Create an Environmentally Friendly Home, by David Pearson, Fireside, NY 1996.

50. ELECTROMAGNETIC FREQUENCIES.

Everything has an electromagnetic field, including us. Our bodies pulse with energy at a frequency of just below 8 hertz while 60 hertz is the level typical of our household electromagnetic fields. Although anything below 300 hertz is considered low frequency radiation, our bodies don't seem to do well with levels much higher than their own. Cancer in children and miscarriage in mothers-to-be are two of the consequences studies attribute to excessive EMF exposure. How much is too much? For the human body, less electricity is always better. Minimizing exposure is the most important step.

The good thing about electromagnetic fields is, the farther you are from them, the more their concentration drops off. However, it's important to remember that *the field is all around the electrical device*, not just in front of it. Electromagnetic radiation emits not just from the front of the television or computer or refrigerator, but also from the sides, top, bottom, and back. If you have a t.v. or computer against one interior wall and there is a bed or couch in the next room against the opposite side of that wall, whoever sleeps or sits there will be radiated whenever the machine is turned on.

In general, it is probably safest to stay three to five feet away from electrical devices. Blow dryers should be held one foot away from the head. Since they are used so briefly and are ineffective at a greater distance, one foot is considered safe. Microwave ovens are best not used, but if you can't live without one, leave the room while it is operating, especially if you have an older model.

Electric blankets are a major source of overexposure, particularly as they tend to be left on all night. Choose not to use them at all, or, turn them on *only* to warm up the bed, then unplug for the night. Same for electric heating pads. These devices may interfere with the body's own electrical patterns. If you need to apply heat to one area of your body, use a hot water bottle.

Keep your head away from a source of electricity. If you use a clock radio for an alarm clock, it should be *a minimum* of three feet away from the pillow or your head receives a steady dose of radiation all night. A clock radio powered with rechargable batteries is a better choice. Avoid sitting too close to an electric light, or attaching a reading lamp to the headboard of your bed where it's right next to your skull. Fluorescent lights are worse than incandescent for radiation. Stay at least six feet away from fluorescent bulbs.

What are the effects on the human body of the network of microwave dishes transmitting phone signals everywhere? There are still many unknowns to the health implications of cordless and cell phones. Anyone who talks on the telephone for extended periods is probably better off to use a regular phone with a cord. This prevents you from having a battery pressed up against your head during your conversations.

However, if you're one of those people who is glued to your cell or cordless phone, you can buy a product called "RayAway". This is a tiny shielding device developed in Scandinavia to protect you from the microwave energy emitted by the phone's antenna. Once you attach it to the receiver, you won't even notice it's there.

In your home, but particularly in your bedroom and your child's play area, turn off and unplug devices when not in use, to lower the amount of electromagnetic radiation. Even when a device is turned off, as long as it is plugged in, the cord is electrified from the wall source.

If you are buying a house, notice where the electric power pylons are located in or near your neighbourhood. These pylons carry massive amounts of electricity and provide a high level of exposure which some studies have linked to childhood leukemia. You will want to be sure your house is a minimum of 500 feet away, and likewise your child's school.

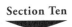

PESTICIDES & LAWN CARE

51. TAKE POISONS SERIOUSLY.

P oison is a strong word. For me, it conjures up images from Agatha Christie and other murder mystery writers. Poison is used on rats, insects, and unfaithful lovers, not on regular people like you and me. Or is it?

Every year, all over the world, billions of pounds of pesticides are manufactured and used in agriculture, apartment buildings, private homes, and public places—schools, offices, parks, and anywhere food is stored or sold—restaurants, shopping centers, grocery stores. Pesticides are poisons.

They linger in buildings, the outdoor environment, the water supply, and in the fatty tissue of your body. No matter where you live, you receive some exposure to these chemicals, whether it's direct exposure from using pesticides, or indirect—from water, foods, and contaminated surfaces.

Pesticides come in three variations: insecticides, herbicides, and fungicides. All three contain both active and "inert" ingredients.

The active ingredient is the actual poison meant to kill insects, plants or fungus. It's usually so toxic it may only represent 1 to 10% of the product. There are perhaps 2,000 so-called "inert" ingredients, including formaldehyde, asbestos, benzene, and phenol, as well as acetone, toluene, and dioxin (the other 1,993 are no picnic either, and it's not easy to get information about them).

In North America since the 1950's, when pesticide use began to take off, there's been an almost magical belief in waging chemical warfare on insects and plants. Pesticides were supposed to be the answer to feeding the world. Over 2 billion pounds per year are used in the U.S. alone. Science author Janine Benyus points out in *Biomimicry* that "crop losses have *increased* 20%" in spite of these megadoses of chemical pesticide!

Pesticide exposure may cause breathing problems, vision impairment, trouble with balance, nausea, skin disorders, memory impairment, neurological disease, depression, heart problems, and damage to internal organs. Between crop losses and the health consequences of pesticides, humans are not faring so well from the practice of waging escalating chemical warfare. Insects, on the other hand, have simply moved on to become "superbugs".

You've probably heard about DDT and its hazardous effects. It's easy to assume that because DDT is no longer used in North America, there's nothing to worry about. Yet DDT is still manufactured and sent to countries that have no ban on its use, and since North Americans often buy produce shipped in from these countries, exposure to DDT residue is quite possible. Also, because of rainfall and weather patterns, any pesticide used *anywhere* in the world can show up in your water supply.

In *Our Stolen Future*, Theo Colborn, Ph.D., points out that the carcinogenic potential of pesticides and other synthetic chemicals is less worrisome than their hormone-disrupting effects. Hormone disruptors interfere with the way brain and physical systems develop in the fetus and young child. There can be impairment of the immune system, alterations in the nervous system or trouble with endocrine development. This can lead to a variety of problems, including increased vulnerability to allergies, attention deficit, behavior and learning disorders, and impaired fertility in adulthood in both men and women. In fact, sperm count seems to be particularly vulnerable to the hormone-scrambling effects of chemicals. A glance at any newspaper shows the number of infertile couples is increasing daily. Coincidence?

We don't actually *know* all the possible effects of synthetic chemicals on the human body, brain, and reproductive system because many chemicals have been tested only for their carcinogenic potential. The few that receive long-term testing are rarely studied beyond the five-year mark, which ignores the effect they may have on the children and later descendents of chemically-exposed parents.

In case you thought a little bit of pesticide was okay but a lot could hurt you, the authors of *Our Stolen Future* point out that hormone disruptors have no respect for amounts. In fact, they can act the *opposite* way from other poisons! In general, the bigger the dose of a toxin, the worse, but in the case of hormone disruptors, a very small dose can have a much more powerful effect! This is particularly true when it hits the body at a crucial developmental point.

In *Eight Weeks to Optimum Health*, Andrew Weil, M.D., mentions a Tulane University study of the estrogenic effects of pesticides. The pesticides alone had limited effects, but when two of them were combined, the effects shot up by several hundred per cent! This study is only one of many indications demonstrating that combinations of pesticides are more dangerous than a single pesticide on its own. Dr. Weil, with other doctors and researchers, advises that pesticides are strongly implicated in the upsurge in breast cancer.

Pesticides are as dangerous as detergents for household poisonings and have a good chance of being fatal. Many household poisonings are caused by pesticides, sometimes because a lawn or garden product is put into an old soft drink bottle or other innocent-looking container, from which a child accidentally drinks. I once believed most pesticides were used out in the country on farmer's fields, however, farmers actually use less pesticide, acre for acre, than homeowners do inside their houses and on their lawns!

When pesticides are sprayed either indoors or on the lawn, you are usually told you can return to the site after a few hours. This advice may be appropriate for a fit, healthy young man, but will the pesticides have dissipated enough for children, pets, pregnant women or *anyone with a compromised immune system* to be in contact with the sprayed surfaces? People with compromised immunity include asthmatics, many of the elderly, and anyone with chronic conditions, heart conditions, or allergies.

Any product with the ending "cide" in its name or a skull and crossbones on the label is a poison. To keep your poison exposure as low as possible and prevent the poisoning of your children and pets, buy organically-grown food, drink filtered water, and don't use pesticides in your house or on your lawn. The next chapter contains lots of ideas for living pesticide-free.

52. SIMPLE AND HEALTHY WAYS TO BUG-OFF.

To keep yourself as safe as possible from these poisons, eliminate, avoid, and reduce! With all the pesticides currently present in the environment, the water system, and the food supply, it's vital to reduce direct and indirect exposure in your home and community.

The first and best step, as with other toxic household chemicals, is to go through your house, garage, and shed and collect every pesticide you come across for disposal at the toxic waste site. These toxins cannot be thrown away with the regular garbage. Look for mothballs, lawn and garden chemicals, household insect sprays and liquids, mouse and rat poisons, lice and flea shampoos, and flea treatments for carpets and upholstery.

Practice caution if you employ such pest professionals as chemical lawn-care services or in-home exterminators. People who do this work may or may not have training or understand the precautions necessary when using pesticides. Regardless of their training level, they are spraying your home or lawn with poisons that have serious health consequences.

Professionals may tell you their products are registered, but registration with a government agency is no guarantee of safety. Factors other than human health and safety figure into the registration process. Chemicals tend to be tested for human safety based on how the average adult male would react, without considering the more sensitive response of a baby, child, pregnant woman, elderly person, or person with health concerns.

Discuss with your neighbours the possibility of making your street a pesticide-free zone. If you happen to like songbirds, a pesticide-free neighbourhood will help to restore our rapidly dwindling bird populations. Birds are the natural predators of insects.

Because chemical warfare is inefficient, management of pests and organic treatment of lawn and garden are better strategies. (Pesticides on foods are a health issue explored in more detail in later chapters.)

Most insects are not harmful to humans and, despite those bad science fiction movies we've all seen, bugs are not out to get you nor do they have any serious plans for taking over the planet. In fact there are lots of insects who are extremely useful, helping out with pollination, without which we'd have no food, killing mosquitoes and flies, breaking down vegetable matter into soil components, and providing food for birds. Unfortunately, these useful insects, like honeybees and ladybirds, may be even more vulnerable to pesticides than the targeted plants and bugs.

Chemical pesticides ultimately make the target insects stronger while doing in the rest of life as we know it—bird, animal, and human. Our culture has perfectionistic standards when it comes to nature—no bugs, no weeds, EVER! Millions of advertising dollars are spent to enforce this concept and convince us the only solution is a chemical one.

As with chemical pesticides, natural methods of pest management will not be *perfect*. They may not work instantaneously. However, they will be *mostly* effective, they won't harm your health and that of your children and pets, they won't force the targeted insects to evolve into superbugs requiring ever higher doses of toxic poisons, and they won't linger in your house for 20 or 30 years, slowly poisoning everyone who lives there.

Here are some suggestions for dealing with the indoor pests in your life. (No, we don't know if they'll work on your boss.) Weeds and outdoor insect repellents are covered in other chapters.

In general:

Here's a safe, easy way to take care of single bugs like flying insects who inadvertantly blunder into your home and want to get out again (which is why they hurl themselves at the windows).

Grab a glass and a piece of heavy paper or lightweight cardboard. A recipe or birthday card is great. Wait for the bug to land on a window or wall or other flat surface, then place the glass over it, being careful not to damage wings or legs. Keeping the glass against the surface, lift one side the tiniest bit so you can carefully slide the cardboard over the mouth of the glass. The cardboard now provides a lid, with the bug trapped inside the glass. Holding the "lid" down, take the whole thing outdoors, lift the lid and let the bug fly away.

This works well with wasps, bees, moths, flies, and so forth. Wasps and bees will not sting you through the cardboard, nor will they rush at you to inflict pain once you release them outdoors. Usually, the insect is so happy to be set free, it flies away as fast as possible. If you're afraid to take the lid off the glass because there's a wasp in it, just set the whole thing down outdoors and run back inside. The breeze will blow the cardboard off and release the bug, then you can reclaim your glass and card.

Ants:

Ants are practical. They are attracted to food. The easiest way to keep ants out of your house is to be sure there is no place for them to enter. Seal up little holes and cracks. And don't give them any incentive to come in.

Instead of storing cereal, cookies, and other food in cardboard boxes and paper bags, put it into glass jars, or keep bags of food inside metal tins or stoneware crocks. In my grandmother's time, people sometimes had a kitchen cupboard that was lined with tin to keep the bugs out. Don't leave crumbs or spills on the kitchen counter or table where you eat, and clear away pets' bowls immediately after their meal.

If ants do come in, despite these precautions, watch them to see where they are entering and seal up that entrance. If it's a door sill or other spot that can't be completely sealed, sprinkle a line of red chile pepper and/or paprika across the sill. Ants will not cross it. I've tried this in my own house and watched the ants turn away in frustration as they encounter the hot spice. After a while, they give up, and life goes on as usual. The great thing about this method is that it cannot harm your pets or children if they get it on their skin or eat it.

For really persistent ants already in your house, make an ant trap by mixing borax with a little water and honey. Mix this up in the bottom of a jar or one of those plastic containers you're clearing out of your house. Put the container near the ants and give them a way to get into it, either by leaning a popsicle stick or other small stick against it as a ramp, or by scrunching masking tape on the outside of the jar for footholds. It may take a day or so for the ants to figure out it's there, but once they do, lots of them will head for this free food and never come out again. Be careful your child or pet does not have access to this container, since borax should not be taken internally. If you prefer, you can buy natural ant bait and borax-based ant traps by mail order from Healthy Home Services.

Or you can sprinkle diatomacheous earth in the area where the ants tend to congregate or the place they enter your house so they must walk across it. You may have to wait a couple of days before the ants go away completely.

Diatomacheous earth is not earth in the sense of garden soil. It looks like fine white powder, and is mined from the compacted fossil remains of diatoms in ancient sea beds. Diatoms were once algae. This white "earth" is completely nontoxic to mammals as there are no chemicals or other harmful substances in it, but it is devastating to insects. For them, it is like walking on glass shards. When they cross it, it cuts their outer shell and they go away and die. Not pleasant, but certainly no worse than chemical sprays, and a million times safer for you and me. Buy it at a natural products store. Do *not* use the kind for swimming pools.

Cockroaches:

Diatomacheous earth is so effective, one natural products store told me the main reason people buy it is for cockroaches. Sprinkle the earth along baseboards and around or under fridges and stoves. Keep surfaces clean. Cockroaches do not actually pose a health problem to humans, but they're unappealing house guests. They are mostly looking for food, so don't give them the opportunity to find it.

Moths:

Mothballs contain paradichlorobenzene, and benzenes are carcinogenic.

There was a time when houses were built with cedar cupboards for seasonal clothing storage. Before that, people used cedar-lined chests to keep their clothes moth-free. Moths hate cedar, and aren't fond of lavendar, mint or bay leaves either, so you can put these herbs in between your sweaters to keep the bugs out.

Clothes should be stored clean, since moths are fond of those little food spots. When storing clothes in a drawer, make sachets from one or all of the herbs listed above or simply twist herbs into a bit of tissue paper and tuck them into the clothes. Or you can go to a pet store and buy the cedar shavings sold to line hamster and guinea pig cages. Put a layer of shavings in the bottom of the drawer and cover with tissue paper. Put the clothes on top of this, then another layer of tissue paper, with cedar shavings on top of that, and voila! You have your own miniature cedar chest.

If you are hanging clothes in a closet, you can tie bags of herbs or cedar shavings to the hanger of each item. Arrange it so the bag hangs down low enough to be among the folds of the clothing, scenting the clothes rather than the hanger.

People who are sensitive to tree turpins will probably want to go with herbs rather than cedar. You may be sensitive to tree turpins if you get sick in February or March (when the sap is running in trees—you may not actually have a cold, but an intolerant reaction) or feel tired, spaced out or high after eating maple syrup.

Fleas:

According to my vet, fleas spend 90% of their time in your carpets and only 10% on your pet. She thinks it makes more sense to treat the house rather than the pet, and I agree with her. It's very hard on pets to be washed with shampoos full of flea-killing toxic chemicals and to wear chemical flea collars on a regular basis, just as it would be hard on us.

Fleas typically go after easy targets—animals who are very young with developing immune systems, old, sick, or with weakened immune systems or acidic blood from a poor diet. The one time our pets had fleas, we had broadloom, so, following our vet's advice, we treated it and left the pets alone. The fleas rapidly disappeared, never to return. (A few years later, the carpets went too, once I learned about their health hazards.)

You can help your pets to be more "flea-rejecting" by improving their diets with fish oils to provide essential fatty acids—this does a wonderful job of eliminating doggie dry skin and dandruff and will give your pet a beautiful shiny coat. Nutritional yeast such as engevita or brewer's yeast to provide B vitamins and bone meal for calcium will help as well. Like mosquitoes, fleas do not like garlic, so feed it to your pets in fresh or powdered form, mixed into their food. Garlic is an immune booster, so will make your pet healthier.

Chemical flea collars release their pesticide over time and these toxins are absorbed into your pet's skin and bloodstream. Flea collars made with herbal repellents rather than chemicals can be found at stores selling natural foods or environmental products as well as some pet suppliers. If your pet is healthy and has no fleas, he or she should not need a flea collar of any sort.

If you do have an infestation of fleas, buy diatomaceous earth (*not* the kind used in swimming pools) to sprinkle on your carpets and pets' bedding. Leave it there as long as you can (all day would be good, but a few hours may do it—and keep your pet off his bed while it's covered with the powdered earth so the fleas won't jump onto him), then vaccuum off. Because fleas jump, it's a little more difficult to get them to walk across the diatomaceous earth than ants or cockroaches, so the longer you can leave it down, the better. The process may have to be repeated a week or so later if the fleas have laid eggs that hatch.

This may seem to you a lot of work, but back in the olden days before I became chemical-wise I used flea bombs once or twice. By the time I had followed the instructions to cover everything in the house that could be damaged or destroyed by the pesticide, gone out for several hours while it did its nasty work, and then come back and cleaned everything up, it would have been *much* easier just to sprinkle some diatomaceous earth. And no toxic residues to live with.

Fruit Flies:

Fruit flies are attracted to vinegar. Make a trap for them by half-filling a jar with any kind of vinegar (white vinegar is fine). Stir in a spoonful of borax, and leave the jar open in a place where the fruit flies gather. It may take a week or ten days for them all to drown themselves, but they will. This is not an instant method, but I know from experience that it works.

While waiting for the fruit flies to commit suicide-by-vinegar, keep your kitchen and house very clean of food scraps and crumbs. Don't leave out anything they can eat. Leave pet food out only long enough for your pet to eat, then refrigerate any leftovers between meals. Store fruit in the fridge (even bananas, just until the flies are gone), and put your compost directly outdoors or keep a small covered container for it in the fridge. A small mixing bowl covered with a plate works well.

If your regular compost bucket has what looks like tiny long thin seed pods on the inside or outside, those are fruit flies getting ready to hatch. Clean your bucket thoroughly and, depending on the time of year, leave out in the full sun or freezing cold for a day. Unless this bucket fits in your fridge, do not use it again until all the fruit flies are dead. If you see any of the "pods" or casings again, clean the bucket immediately to prevent them from hatching.

Spiders:

Spiders create such panic, the first reaction many people have is to grab the nearest blunt object and squash the little beasts. In spite of Little Miss Muffet and Arachnophobia, the humble spider deserves better.

There are many varieties of spider that do not harm humans, unless you live in Australia where, according to travel writer Bill Bryson, practically everything that moves can kill you. Except, maybe, the kangaroos. Spiders are good at killing bugs like flies and mosquitoes. Before you flatten the next spider you see, check a book on spiders to find out whether your little housemate is dangerous (more typical in southern areas) or phone the poison centre and ask what poisonous spiders look like.

Even if yours is not a threat to human health, you may prefer to have it out of your living space. Take a glass or jar and put it over the spider. Quickly slide a piece of paper or an index card under the glass, trapping the spider inside, and take it out of doors to be set free. That way the spider can still kill flying bugs outside for you.

And then read *Charlotte's Web*. You'll feel a lot better about spiders afterwards.

Mice:

One of the dangers of chemical mouse poison, particularly the kind you set out in dishes or spread in cupboards, is that your pets and/or young children can get into it and either eat it or lick it off their paws.

As with ants, it's important to seal up holes and make sure there is no way for mice to get into your house, and no available food to tempt them. The number one most effective exterminator of mice is a cat. The ancient Egyptians worshipped cats, no doubt in part because cats protected the valuable stores of world-famous Egyptian grain from rodents. If you don't want a cat of your own, borrow one from a friend for a few days.

If you or family members are allergic to cats, buy and set some good old-fashioned mousetraps. If you have toddlers or pets, be sure to place them out of reach of fingers, paws, and noses. Mousetraps are probably more humane than glue-type traps since, when they are set and baited correctly, they will kill the mouse outright, instead of forcing it through a sticky, painful, and lingering death.

For more information, read:
Least Toxic Home Pest Control by Dan Stein, The Book Publishing Co., Summertown, TN, 1994.

53. GRASS. HOW GREEN SHOULD IT BE?

Lawns are monocultures—the planting of a single species over a broad area. Nature *never* grows this way. Monocultures are notoriously difficult to maintain, are hard on the soil, invite pest infestations, and are not naturally self-sustaining.

Unlike Nature, we import monocultures to climates where they do not belong, for example, planting green lawns in the desert environment of Nevada where they require unnatural (for the geography) amounts of water. Even in a temperate zone, a green lawn is something of an anomaly to the natural world. So why are we obsessed with cultivating these manicured plateaus of green?

In the 1800's, lawn games became popular, and short grass was needed for golf, bowling, tennis, and croquet. An expanse of green lawn would have been achievable only by the affluent (who else would have time for tennis and golf?) and therefore carried the glamor of other elite possessions.

Ironically, *grass pollens and turpins* (the juice of cut grass) *are major allergens* affecting thousands of adults and children. With that and the millions of pounds of synthetic fertilizer and pesticides poisoning us, our passion for lawns has backfired on us.

Can you achieve an outdoor carpet of brilliant green without chemical pesticides and fertilizers? Yes, if you're willing to have a mixture of species on your lawn, otherwise probably not. Grass has a natural cycle. When the season is hot and dry, grass naturally turns brown, conserving itself to turn green again in autumn rains.

Chemical lawns manage their continual pop-up green look through high levels of nitrogen in the fertilizer. This type of fertilizer, along with regular doses of synthetic herbicide and fungicide, offers no micronutrients and tends to disrupt the soil ecosystem, eradicating earth worms and microbial activity which would otherwise help to keep grass healthy.

The chemical lawn is vulnerable—just as we are when our bodies are overloaded with toxins—and easily stressed. When a grub infestation or other problem comes along, the chemical lawn has no resources to deal with it. Organic lawns, on the other hand, are resilient and pest-resistant. Pests will pass over the organic lawn in favor of the easy target already weakened by chemicals. I've seen this happen in my own neighbourhood. My next-door neighbour's lawn, after years of chemicals, is regularly dug up by night-prowlers seeking grubs, while our organic lawn is left untouched.

I spoke to an organic lawn expert and learned that untreated lawns have all the nutrients they need to cope with the seasons on their own. She listed three typical mistakes we all make with our lawns:

1) *Cutting the grass too short.* Cutting grass short stresses the lawn and allows weed seeds to germinate! Only the top 1/3 of a blade of grass should be cut, or the plant goes into shock, which increases its vulnerability to pests. Grass needs to be about three inches high to promote root growth and crowd out weed seeds. A thick, healthy lawn will not allow weeds room to grow.

2) *Overwatering.* Most of us water our lawns far too much. The maximum a lawn needs is one hour a week of good watering that soaks the

roots (except under rare circumstances like drought). Healthy lawns in zones where there is occasional rainfall can usually be left without any watering at all. Frequent shallow watering—watering the grass lightly—promotes weak root growth.

3) *Using too many chemicals.* When we do use chemicals, we tend to overdo it. Then the lawn becomes dependent on chemicals, because they're the only thing propping it up. Breaking away to a lawn nurtured by nature rather than synthetically-derived additives means giving the grass and soil a little time to make the transition, but it also means less labor and expense (not to mention fewer toxins).

Surprising as it sounds, just leaving your lawn alone and cutting it to a height of about 3 inches is the simplest and most organic route to a healthy lawn. If you want to help it along a little, leave the grass cuttings on the lawn. They are a wonderful source of natural—as opposed to synthetically derived—nitrogen. You can have your lawn aerated, or you can overseed it (put down lots of grass seed) to crowd out weeds. If you do get the occasional unwanted weed, hand weed, then overseed the turned up earth.

Some people with organic lawns encourage weeds so they can collect free dandelion leaves to put in salads for an excellent source of calcium. Others prefer weeds because they attract certain bird species. Another term for weeds is "naturally occuring native species." You may decide you enjoy the variety these natural species provide to your lawn.

54. CHOOSING FERTILIZERS AND LAWN CARE COMPANIES.

ertilizers come in an N-P-K formula: nitrogen, phosphorus, and potassium, reflected by three numbers on the package. Synthetically derived fertilizers with their high water-solubility will have numbers like 10-6-4, or 21-7-7. The high first number indicates a large dose of nitrogen meant to jolt your lawn quickly into total greenness, then it exhausts your soil. Chemically derived fertilizer provides no micronutrients for plants and is highly *water-soluble.* If you apply it right before a rainfall or before watering your lawn, more than 50% washes away into the water system where you drink it.

Organic compilations are slow release, and have much lower numbers, like 6-4-4. Garden centers that are unfamiliar with organic methods may tell you that the N-P-K numbers are so low, you have to use three times as much! Don't believe them.

Read labels carefully. *A product that's 100% organic should say so on the package.* However, sewage sludge is 100% organic, so if you're uncomfortable with that, check the package for information about ingredient sources. What you *don't* want in your fertilizer are urea, ammonia, potassium chloride or muriate of potassium.

Organic ingredients include soy, which is vegetable source, as well as animal sources: poultry manure, feather meal, turkey compost, composted cow manure, and leather. If leather is an ingredient, heavy metals (arsenic, cadmium, etc.) or chemical additives in the leather may be a concern. Composting usually removes pathogens so when animal materials are listed as being composted, they are probably okay. (Feather meal won't be composted.) The lower on the food chain fertilizer ingredients are, the fewer toxins they contain. Vegetable or plant matter is low on the food chain. Animal is high.

Your own compost from vegetable matter and leaves contains micronutrients and will help to improve soil structure, particularly when you take your lawn off chemicals. You can mix it with water and pour it on, or just spread or sprinkle it.

When composting your kitchen scraps, cut up large, thick items like flower stems or celery stalks and skins from banana, melon, citrus fruit or squash. Smaller, thinner pieces break down faster than large pieces. Do not include animal products—milk, yogurt, butter, fat, meat or large bones. Some people do put in chicken bones and fish skin—fish is often a fertilizer ingredient. *Do* put in egg shells, coffee grounds, and tea bags or leaves.

In the kitchen, plastic buckets for compost scraps will absorb and preserve stinky odors. The only way to get the smell out is to use a toxic chlorine bleach, or to buy endless replacements. I prefer an enamel bucket with its own lid. The enamel does not absorb odors, is easy to clean, petrochemical-free, and will probably last me the rest of my life. Kitchen or hardware stores carry enamel buckets.

When looking for a lawn care service with natural or organic methods, here are some guidelines to keep in mind:

1) *Are any chemical fertilizers, pesticides, or herbicides used?* If the prospective company answers this by saying, "Don't worry," that's not good enough. They should be able to tell you if there are chemicals being used in any format.

One of the chemicals for lawn care is 2,4-D, a mixture also found in Agent Orange, the herbicide used in Vietnam and linked to cancers that occured many years later in veterans of that war as well as congenital problems in their children. 2,4-D can be and often is contaminated with dioxin. Needleman and Landrigan, authors of *Raising Children Toxic Free*, plainly state, "Dioxin [is] the most toxic synthetic chemical known."

Many companies use a granular pesticide formula for grub control. This formula contains Diazinon. Although this poison kills birds, cannot be used on golf courses, sod farms, or corn fields, and is suspected of causing birth defects in humans, it is still okayed for our lawns!

Even more bizarre is that *ninety percent* of what is sprayed on lawns by lawn care companies (or us) does not reach its target because of wind drift, and there doesn't have to be much wind. The lightest puff of air will do it. So the chemical ends up on the flowers in your garden, on lawn furniture and toys, in swimming pools, and on the street, where it cannot be absorbed by the asphalt so it washes down the sewer into the water system. It also kills beneficial insects like ladybirds.

2) *Does the company use terms such as "organic-based", "environmentally friendly", or "natural source"?* Some companies will call their treatment "environmentally friendly" because they spot spray rather than blanket spray chemicals on your lawn! "Organic-based" is another deceptive term. It means there is only a *minimum* of organic ingredients and the rest is chemical.

"Organic pesticides" are derived from an organic source, so they will break down quicker, don't accumulate, and have *low* mammalian toxicity but they do kill beneficial insects. And considering the body's total toxic load, low mammalian toxicity may simply not be good enough. *NO* mammalian toxicity is a much healthier choice.

Labelling a treatment product "natural source" doesn't mean it's safe. After all, arsenic is from a natural source and so is petroleum (the source is natural, the processing is not!) In fact, the chemical definition of an "organic" substance is that it contains carbon. Dioxin contains carbon, hence it could be called organic!

3) *Does the company tell you their products are safe because they are registered (with a government body or official authority)?* Unfortunately, pesticides are not safe just because they're registered. The registration process is based on many factors, only one of which is human safety. Many chemicals are registered with only the most superficial and sometimes outdated testing for their effect on human health. If a company tells you not to worry because their products are registered, don't be fooled.

4) *What does the program entail?* In general, truly organic lawn care companies will *not* use herbicides and pesticides. The organic strategy is to make the lawn so healthy it discourages weeds and pests on its own. (Similar to what you want to do for your body.) Fertilizers or soil amendments from the organic sources listed above (soy, poultry manure, feather meal, composted cow manure, turkey compost) will be used. These products will not endanger the health of children, adults, pets or your local songbirds.

Lawn care companies who use organic or natural methods will aerate or overseed your lawn and keep the grass on the long side to crowd out weeds instead of spraying it with herbicides. Some may provide hand-weeding services, although this is not as important as providing a good program to generate a healthy lawn, especially since some weeds are nature's way of trying to restore nutrients to your lawn. The healthy lawn discourages pests, so there will be no need for pesticides.

If the company provides weekly lawn servicing (cutting), ask if *they* do it, or if they hire someone to do it. You want to know the person cutting your lawn uses good techniques. This means they should not cut your grass too short, as this encourages weed germination, they should not overwater your lawn or tell you to do a lot of watering, except as needed to germinate new grass seed, and they should leave the grass clippings on the lawn to provide nitrogen.

For more information, read:
Natural Lawn Care, by Dick Raymond, Storey Communications Inc., Pownal, VT 1993.

55. LAWN ALTERNATIVES.

Want to free yourself of the whole lawn-care scenario? Consider not having a lawn at all. This sounds like a radical idea in North America, where having a lawn seems an established fact of home ownership.

One of the most beautiful front yards in our neighbourhood has no lawn. Instead, it is a country garden with flowers, flagstones, a couple of trees, and handsome twig chairs for relaxation. A pair of pseudo sheep peek out from amongst the greenery. The effect is charming, inviting, and far more visually interesting than a lawn. Another neighbour with a tiny front yard sews perennial wildflower seeds and plants lilies across it. The effect is gorgeous and the flowers last all season.

Some people grow vegetables or herbs in their front yards. It is estimated that, all over North America where we now have lawns, there is sufficient arable land to grow food crops for the entire population, should we (gulp!) lose all our farm land to housing developments or agricultural disaster. In the midwest, one third of the topsoil, which takes thousands of years to restore itself, has blown away due to monoculture and agribusiness farming practices over the last hundred years.

The organic lawn service I use recommends clover, herb lawns or native grass species as an alternative to the standard lawn of golf course type grass. These alternatives are attractive, unusual, and easy-care. But they do make you rethink your concept of how a lawn ought to look. Instead of a high-tech green carpet, they will look more like a meadow—a little wilder and more natural. They *are* good for your soil, helping to restore nutrients, and may even attract butterflies and songbirds.

If your lawn is more for visual than traffic purposes, or you want to fill in an area with low-maintenance greenery, try a ground cover like perennial thyme which produces a small purple flower, has a nice scent, and makes a dense, springy carpet of green.

Taking Action

56. DISCOVER YOUR LOCAL TOXIC WASTE DUMP.

Have you ever had this thought? "If a product was *that* dangerous, they wouldn't sell it." Guess again. Product availability is no guarantee of safety to your health. Many products cost far more than their retail price because of the extended damage they cause to health, plumbing, and water and sewer systems. So in addition to paying for them through your well-being and medical costs, you pay through your home repair and tax bills and having to purchase safe water. In the 21st century, drinkable water may well incite the same type of international struggle caused by petroleum in the 20th century.

If you put toxic waste into the regular garbage, even when it is in a container inside your garbage bag, sooner or later the bags and containers leak, so the chemicals drain into the soil and then into the water system. This is one of the ways chemicals end up in your drinking water and the food you eat.

The best way to locate the nearest toxic waste dump is to phone your municipal or regional government's waste collection or works department. They can tell you where to find the toxic dump, what hours it keeps, what waste is accepted, and if a pick-up service is available. They may even have some free literature to send you describing hazardous waste and safe alternative products.

The following types of products are classified for toxic waste disposal: paints, solvents, glues, automotive products, pesticides, weed killers, chemical fertilizers, pool chemicals, mothballs, rat and mouse poison, air fresheners, batteries, lighter fluid, chemical household cleaners, and some personal care products such as nail polish remover, perfume, aftershave, and other alcohol-based products.

If you *must* use a toxic product, buy a small amount—just enough for the job you are doing—and use it all up right away. Try to choose environmentally-friendly paints and finishes that require only water clean-up for the brushes or rollers. Instead of pouring the clean-up water down the sink, where it goes straight into the drinking water system, pour it into a container with a lid and take it to the toxic waste dump. If you've almost finished a can of paint, let the paint residue harden in the can—outside or in the garage—and then throw the can into the regular garbage.

As of 2001, all consumer household chemical products were supposed to be labelled for toxicity. Even so, play it safe—if the product has to go to the toxic waste depot for disposal, you probably won't want to bring it into your home or your life in the first place.

57. ORGANIZING THE CHANGES.

Changing your household from old toxic products to new health-supporting ones is simple but it does take some time. You are learning a new skill set, so be gentle with yourself and don't expect to do it overnight. To accomplish the transition you can proceed room by room, by type of toxin or simply by following the chapters in this book and using them as an action plan.

Here are some guidelines for proceeding room by room. Your bedroom is a good place to start, because this is the room you probably spend the most time in. While you sleep, your body has some down time to work at healing and restoring itself from the stresses of the day, whether those stresses are physical, chemical, mental or emotional in nature. If your bedroom is full of toxins, your body has to spend its sleep time coping with those toxins instead of resting and doing vital healing work. So it makes sense that the place where you sleep be as toxin-free as possible.

Clear out scented products, candles, plastics, and room deodorizers. Replace scented and paraffin candles with beeswax or soybean oil candles, or put your paraffin candles out only when in use and store them in a tin or jar the rest of the time. Store books and magazines outside the bedroom and put the current book you are reading into a drawer overnight. If you are mold-sensitive or have any type of breathing problem, move plants and aquariums to another room.

Instead of synthetic broadloom, have sealed wood or ceramic tile floors with washable cotton throw rugs, or wool carpets. Seal particle board furniture with wood sealer. Use cotton thermal or wool blankets, quilts stuffed with cotton, silk or poly fibers instead of feathers, and pillows filled with cotton or poly fiber, wool batting or buckwheat hulls. Wash clothes and bedding with safe laundry products. Hang dry-cleaned clothes in a room where no one sleeps and look for a "green" (non-toxic) dry cleaner.

After the bedroom, work on the room where you spend the most time. For some people this will be the kitchen. Check for toxic cleaners, plastic bags, plastic wrap and other soft plastics, room deodorizers, improperly vented gas stoves, unsealed particle board cupboards or furniture, and broadloom. Gas stoves should be vented to the outdoors. Avoid natural gas if anyone in the house has asthma.

You can then move on to the other rooms: living room, bathrooms, laundry room, and so forth, using this book as a guide to show you what to clear out.

Another way to take action is to proceed through the house by type of toxin. This is an easy way to work if you have a limited amount of time to spare for making changes. Begin, for example, with paints, oils, and solvents. Take a box with you and quickly check over the whole house for these problem substances. You probably know where most of them are, but check your closets anyway, in case you're like a friend of mine who discovered a large can of turpentine outgassing in her coat cupboard! Put the box in the garage or storage shed for future use or delivery to the toxic waste dump.

When you next have some available time, clear your house of plastic bags and put those you need into tins. After that, work on fragranced products, exchanging new, toxin-free, and unscented ones for old chemical versions. You might begin by changing your laundry and personal care products, move on to dish and household cleaners, and eliminate room deodorizers and other unnecessary sources of chemical scent. Then, source good bottled drinking water or a possible filter system to go into your home. And so forth.

Longer term projects which involve some planning and a little extra time include taking out broadloom and installing health-supporting flooring, sealing furniture and particle board kitchen cabinets, and installing a water filter system. These are changes that usually have to wait until time and finances are in place. You may also find you need time to adapt psychologically to these changes. Until the changes are in place, it's easy to underestimate their benefits to your well-being.

The sooner you can clear the worst toxins out of your house and create a pollution-free haven, the easier life will be for your immune system. When your body is no longer struggling with toxins in your home, you will have increased energy and time for making other health-supporting changes. It took years to develop your current lifestyle habits, and it can easily take a year or more to organize a health-supporting way of life. So give yourself lots of time.

And do the things that are easiest for you first. If you're not ready to change a particular aspect of your life, begin with something you *are* willing to alter. For example, if you're very attached to a particular food even though you suspect it may not be that good for you, focus on eliminating the chemical toxins from your home. A toxin-free house will help reduce your total toxic load and make it easier for your body to cope with the food. You might also try purchasing the organically-grown, chemical-free version of your favorite food. Every small step you take will add up over the months, contributing long-term benefits to your well-being.

If you have a friend or friends who are interested in making health-supporting changes, start making them together. It's easier and more fun to make these changes with friends, so you can compare notes on the improvements you notice, the difficulties you encounter, the great new products and services you discover, and the best places to buy or access them.

It's more fun to try new things with a friend.

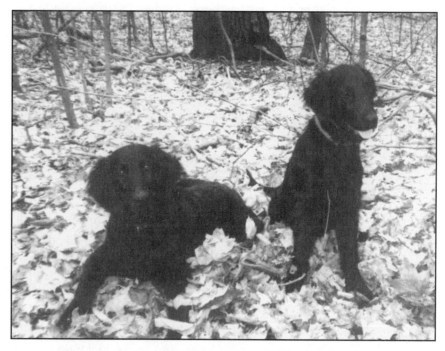

"Mom, we're ready to try out your organic picnic now!"

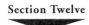

WATER

58. DRINK WATER.

After air, the element most important to human life and well-being is water. Water is vital to almost every bodily process. You can live for about a month and a half without food, but without water you die in less than a week!

Brain function, healing, digestion, breathing, clearing out toxins, weight regulation, blood volume, blood pressure regulation, skin quality, and many other processes utilize water in one way or another. Dr. F. Batmanghelidj, author of *Your Body's Many Cries for Water*, presents powerful evidence to show that many chronic conditions and diseases come about because of dehydration. He cites lack of adequate water as a contributing factor in morning sickness, asthma, digestive disorders, kidney trouble, constipation, peptic ulcers, back pain, dry skin, hypertension, excess cholesterol, arthritis, headaches, depression, sleep disturbances, overweight, bulimia, and allergies.

Dehydration is not well understood. I used to think I was thirsty if my mouth felt dry. Then I learned a dry mouth is a sign of advanced dehydration! The solution is to drink water regularly during the day without waiting for a thirst signal from your body.

Lots of us misinterpret the thirst signal, anyway. According to Dr. Batmanghelidj, thirst is often mistaken for hunger or tiredness. If you eat instead of drinking water, you end up dehydrating your body further and you may continue feeling cravings because your body is seeking water, not food! The best thing to do before responding to your snack attack is to drink a glass of water, *then* eat. Tiredness and headaches are sometimes a sign of dehydration. If you feel a slump around four in the afternoon, drink some water.

No substitute answers your body's need for water. Caffeinated beverages are diuretic and cause further dehydration. Juice, milk, and other drinks are processed by the body as food and provide little in the way of hydration. Herbal teas are okay as water sources some of the time, but because herbs are the basis of many medications, it's best not to drink them all day.

Most authorities recommend six to eight 8-ounce glasses of pure, clean water *every day* to keep your body functioning efficiently and in a disease-free state. In case you're worried that all this water will have you spending half the day in the bathroom, you may be surprised to find water stimulates your kidneys and bladder far less than caffeinated beverages. Besides being diuretic, caffeine can register in your body as a toxin to be excreted as fast as possible.

CAUTION! If you haven't been drinking much water, don't start with eight glasses! I did this, not knowing any better, and felt terrible at first. I began to wonder if I had some unsuspected disease or had suddenly developed high blood pressure. It passed after a few days, but it was extremely frightening and uncomfortable. Luckily for me, I survived my water binge. I wouldn't recommend it to anyone else!

A healthier way is to start with a couple of glasses a day and build up the amount of water you drink slowly over two or three weeks, gradually replacing your other beverages with water. Be particularly careful if you have any heart or circulatory problems. The water will do you good, unless you try to reach maximum intake overnight like I did!

59. IMPROVE YOUR WATER.

If you've seen a photograph of Earth from space, you know that her predominant color is blue. Most of our planet is covered with water, however, only about 3% of this water is usable by humans! The other 97% is salt water. And of the usable fresh water, 75% is frozen in glaciers!

Imagine going through a single day without water. How would you shower, wash your hands, brush your teeth, do dishes or laundry, prepare food and cook, or give yourself or your pets a drink? It would be a nightmare!

Since water is so important and there seems to be so little available for human use, you'd think we would do everything possible to safeguard it. Yet our precious water supply is in big trouble from pollutants.

Water pollution is not cleared up by municipal water treatment, which mostly filters out sediment from human waste and tries to eliminate bacteria through chlorination. Municipalities do not allot funds to filter for industrial and agricultural pollutants—the technology for this is expensive. Water is also polluted by leaks from underground gas and oil tanks, radiation and viruses, not all of which are killed by municipal treatment plants.

A huge amount of raw sewage in North America comes from livestock. In fact, meat and dairy animals use up far more water than humans do— more than 50% of all potable water goes to animal farming! Producing *one* beef cow takes 1.2 million gallons of water.

Since livestock and industry are busy polluting the water while competing with the rest of us for the 3% of water that is drinkable, we need some protection! Here are some steps you can take to ensure your household supply of water is not contaminated.

Use filtered water:

Filtering water requires a better system than a jug with a little throw-away filter in it. For one thing, these filtering jugs are not very effective at purifying water. More importantly, you need a good system because the water you wash with affects you as much as the water you drink. Pollutants in your water can be absorbed by your skin when bathing, and you put them in your mouth when brushing your teeth (you can't help swallowing a few molecules). Also, the steam from bath and shower water releases chlorine and other pollutants into the air, so you inhale them.

There are different options for improving your water. You can purchase a whole-house water system, which filters the water where it comes into your house, so that every tap provides good water. Or you can install one filter at the kitchen faucet so you'll have good water for drinking and food preparation, and another in the bathroom directly on the shower head. A third option is to purchase good-quality bottled drinking water, which in many cities can be delivered regularly to your house at a nominal cost, and, again, put a chlorine-removing filter on the shower head.

When choosing the second or third options, use filtered or bottled water when you brush your teeth and not the water straight from the bathroom tap, otherwise you'll ingest the very contaminants you're trying to avoid! Once you have begun to filter the water in your home, be sure to take some with you to drink when you go out.

Types of purification systems:

There are basically three types of water purifier: active charcoal (or activated carbon), reverse osmosis, and steam distillation. The last two have proven in lab tests to be the most effective at decontaminating water, however, the purification system that will get *everything* out of your water has not yet been invented. If you live in a rural area, add an ultra violet filter or boil your water to kill bacteria.

If you are considering a home system, you may want to have your household water tested by an outside agency to determine what contaminants need to be removed. Your choice of systems will also depend on what level of convenience you prefer. Although distillation is considered to remove the highest level of contaminants, it is also the most labour-intensive method and takes about seven parts water to make one part distilled water. (e.g. seven litres or quarts of tap water make one litre or quart of distilled water.)

Neither reverse osmosis nor steam distillation remove chlorine from water. If you live in a chlorinating municipality, you can either boil your filtered water before drinking it, add a charcoal filter to remove chlorine, or simply fill a pitcher and allow it to sit for a couple of hours before drinking. The chlorine will evaporate.

Before you make your choice of a water filter system, read Consumer Reports, talk to friends, visit health fairs, and ask lots of questions of water-filter dealers. Ask what their system does, whether it has removable or replaceable parts and, if so, how often they need replacement, how long the company has been in business, what literature they can give you about their product, what their replacement policy is in case of malfunction and so forth. It's like buying any other appliance.

If you are not in a position to spend money on changing your water, you can take the following temporary measures.

1) Lead can accumulate in water sitting in pipes overnight. To reduce levels of lead, run the water for at least 90 seconds before using. Do not cook with water heated by the hot water tap. Follow the same principle in a public building, especially if you are the first one in in the morning—let the water run before drinking or using it.

2) Avoid drinking fountains. They are often contaminated with bacteria. Encourage your children to bring their own bottled drinking water from home rather than drinking from school water fountains. In these days of designer bottled waters, it's glamorous to tote your own special water!

3) Some pollutants can be removed by boiling your drinking water for ten minutes, preferably in a glass or stainless steel pot, and allowing it to cool before using. Nancy Sokol Green warns that while this will take out chlorine, pesticides, and bacteria, it will not remove trace minerals, heavy metals, or organic chemicals. There is some concern that these substances may even be concentrated by boiling, however, this method is probably better than doing nothing at all.

4) The ultraviolet rays of the sun kill bacteria. Put water in a clear (not colored) glass bottle or jug and leave in direct sunlight for five hours.

Kathy and I have both worked with people who made significant improvements in their health once they improved the water they were using in their daily lives. One man with bowel problems told me he reduced his symptoms by 75 to 80% after he installed a water filtration system in his house!

Swimming pools:

Instead of using chemicals in your pool water, try salt. A salt water pool feels wonderful on the skin and is easier and less expensive to maintain (since you will not need weekly testing and gallons of chemicals). Even your dog can swim in a salt water pool. You will need to have a salinator installed. Sometimes it's difficult to find a pool company to do this, since salt water pools are still new to some areas. The average system uses around 3,000 parts per million (ppm) salt concentration. I have read that the ideal is about 9,000 ppm, while the ocean averages closer to 33,000 ppm. You can research this on the internet by looking up salt water pools.

For more information, read:
Don't Drink the Water (without reading this book) The Essential Guide to Our Contaminated Drinking Water and What You Can Do About It, by Lono Kahuna Kapua A'o, Kali Press, Pagosa Springs, CO 1996.

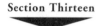

Food in General

60. RETHINK YOUR DEFINITION OF FOOD.

What *is* food? I used to think of it as anything I liked the taste of—potato chips, chicken, cookies, apples, raisins, chocolate bars, ice cream, salad, bacon—it was all food to me. Then I started to learn about food processing, chemicals, and their effects on mental, physical, and emotional health. All of a sudden, a lot of things I once called "food" switched into a whole other category as I realized those items were robbing me of nutrients and filling me up with pollutants.

Now I define food as something that offers me nourishment. That doesn't mean it's boring—the best food is always fun to eat, not only because it tastes so good, but because it makes you feel great after you eat it.

And that's another important aspect of food. I learned the long and painful way that what I put into my body determined how I felt afterwards. The right foods make me feel energetic, lively, focussed, content, able, strong, and coordinated. The wrong foods made me irritable, sleepy, hungry with cravings, anxious, gassy, disoriented, forgetful, uncomfortable, crampy, and whiny.

Some of the foods I thought I liked most, like sugary sweets and other junk foods, turned out not to be my favorites after all. I ate them repetitively in an attempt to balance my neurotransmitters, boost my energy level, and upgrade my emotional state. I've since discovered how to do these things through whole foods, which provide good nutrition and none of the negative side effects of sweets and caffeine. Candace Pert, Ph.D., points out that the less you seek "highs" from sugar, alcohol, caffeine, and other stimulants, the more your body will produce its own energy-boosting peptides.

Despite the many variations of "junk" food available, most of them contain a selection from the same few ingredients: wheat, corn, sugar, salt, fat, caffeine, and dairy. Look at any processed food on the shelf and you'll find one or more of these typical components, as well as preservatives and flavors derived from petrochemicals and colors made from coal tar! Perhaps not so surprisingly, this list of convenience and junk food ingredients includes six of the most common allergens (wheat, corn, sugar, caffeine, dairy, and chemicals).

Since I now think of food as nourishment, I notice much of what is available on the shelves of the grocery store is *not* what I would define as food. In general, the more processing a food product receives, the less nutrition it contains. Grocery store food products containing unpronounceable ingredients tend to be loaded with chemicals, colors, flavors, sweeteners, and cooked fats that do nothing good for the human body. These packaged foods have a long shelf life—they can sit around for months but are kept from tasting as stale and rancid as they really are with preservatives.

Many people think of food as calories, but calories are only a measure of heat and tell you nothing about the real value of the food to your body. One chocolate chip cookie has five fewer calories than a cup of parsley. According to the caloric theory of eating, this would make it a better choice for someone who wants to reduce their calories. But the cookie contains little nutrition whereas the parsley is loaded with vitamins, minerals, fiber, a little protein and water, and makes a great salad. Instead of calories, it is probably more useful to think of food in terms of the nutrients it provides.

Nutrients—what the body needs to perform its functions and keep you healthy and happy—are found in protein foods, vegetables, fruit, nuts, seeds, and high-quality oils. This short list, which contains tremendous variety when you look at all the foods it encompasses, is what I've come to think of as food. Food is the stuff that actually makes your body *work properly* and *feel good*.

In the following chapters, we are going to look at foods that add to your health, foods that don't, and ways to eat healthier without buying *everything* from the natural foods store.

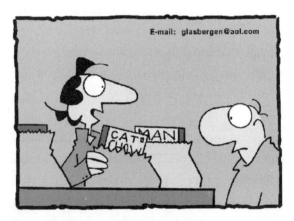

"This new store has simplified everything.
All they sell is Dog Chow, Cat Chow,
Man Chow, Woman Chow and Kid Chow."

61. EAT FOR NUTRIENT VALUE.

Eating for nutrient value might sound a little obvious. Don't we all know we're supposed to do that, already? Well, yes and no.

If you're a typical North American, eating for nutrient value is a pretty radical notion. Like me, you probably grew up valuing food for many reasons that had little to do with nutrition. In my teens and twenties, nutrition was an abstract notion—it meant eating daily from the four food groups: Chocolate, Sugar, Ice cream and Other foods. (Does this sound familiar?) The idea of food actually becoming my *cells* never occurred to me.

Until I noticed I wasn't feeling that great!

So what does eating for nutrient value mean? It means choosing foods that give you the maximum boost for each bite. The nutrient value of foods depends on various factors, including how and where the food was grown, how much it's been processed, and how it's cooked. Foods grown in denatured soil offer you little in the way of nutrition. Even so, a vegetable or fruit grown in denatured soil will offer more than a food product made with stabilizers, preservatives, cooked and altered fats, bleached flour and sugar, and irradiated spices. Fried, deep-fried, and burnt foods are toxic.

When a food stresses your immune system, you can have difficulty absorbing its nutrients. The top food allergens can cause problems for *everyone* whether or not you have allergies. They include dairy, wheat, corn, sugar, and caffeine (chocolate, soft drinks, coffee, black tea), as well as peanuts, yeast, oranges and orange juice, eggs, pork (bacon, ham, luncheon meats, etc.), shellfish, food additives, and colors. These foods typically contain high levels of pesticides, antibiotics, chemical residues, molds, hybridization, dyes or pollutants which may contribute to their problematic effects.

When I got the chemicals out of my house and switched to eating for nutrient value, here are some of the benefits I experienced. Loss of food cravings and reduced appetite (no doubt because of increased nutrient levels.) Stabilized weight. Balanced emotions, better concentration, and improved sleep. More energy. More stamina, strength, and coordination during physical exercise. Improved digestion. Colds and sickness became rare.

To eat for nutrient value, you don't need a specific diet plan. Instead, consider the following guidelines. Choose whole foods: fruits, vegetables, grains, nuts, seeds, legumes, eggs, low-fat protein foods. Eat protein foods according to your needs (athletes, pregnant women, and growing teens usually need more than sedentary people.) Buy organic as much as possible to avoid chemical residues, irradiation, drugs, and artificial additives. Choose organically-grown chocolate and coffee to reduce your pesticide intake (these are heavily sprayed crops). Avoid allergenic, highly-processed, and junk foods. Read labels when shopping—labels reveal a multitude of information about food products. Eat a wide variety of foods—repetitive eating of the same foods leads to intolerances (stress on the immune system.)

Eat only high quality fats/oils. Run for your life from fried and deep-fried foods, and refined white sugar. Drink plenty of clean water. Make eating choices based on what works best for your body rather than what is dictated by social custom or holiday tradition. Don't worry about making mistakes. Practice gratitude that you have a choice about what you eat.

62. EAT SOMETHING DIFFERENT EVERY DAY.

Do you tend to eat the same foods over and over again? You can survive on monotony, but you'll thrive on variety. By eating a wide variety of foods over several days, your body gets a full range of nutrients. Variety also keeps you from creating food sensitivities or reactions. A peculiarity of the human body is that when you eat the same food over and over again, you can develop a reaction to it. Reactions are tiring, irritating, and stressful and can be an unsuspected source of many health concerns.

It takes about four or five days for a food to completely clear from your body, so if you eat a certain food only once every four to seven days, it's less likely to cause trouble. There are so many foods available, it's easy to figure out an interesting plan or "rotation". A food rotation is when you vary your foods so you eat different ones every day for a week. More about this in the next chapter.

If you *are* going to eat repetitively, which is sometimes unavoidable even with the best intentions, choose good foods and try to buy the best quality. For example, when I'm in a rush, the foods I typically eat over and over again are apples, dried fruit, nuts, baby carrots, cocoa powder (for hot drinks), and Edenblend rice/soy drink. I compensate for this repetitiveness by buying organically-grown versions (Edenblend is an organic product) and making sure I vary my dinners. For me, this is a tremendous improvement over the years when I had a daily dose of ice cream, chocolate chip cookies, and coffee. What do *you* eat over and over again? Even if it's cookies, you can usually find a healthy version that will be easier on your body. In the following chapters, we'll look at ways to make healthier food choices.

63. MAKING A FOOD PLAN.

I'll tell you right now that making a food plan involves some work. You don't have to do it and it's not a prerequisite for good health. But once you get it organized, it does simplify shopping and food preparation since you always know what to buy and what you're going to eat. No more of those frustrating debates about what to have for dinner. The other great thing about a food plan is that it makes it easy to vary your foods and eat lots of different nutrients. After the initial planning effort, you don't have to think about it any more. You just follow the plan.

To make up a food rotation, you need to know that foods belong to different botanical "families". For example, most grains, the basic ingredient in bread, pasta, cereal, and baked goods, belong to the Grass Grain family. You can find out about food families by phoning your local allergy association, or from a library book containing food family tables. These are often in books about dietary allergies.

An easy way to plan your rotation is to think in terms of categories: protein, vegetables, fruit, grains, calcium sources. A meal should include foods from at least two categories. You also need to like what you're eating. Try to have a little protein in one form or another at every meal, plus a couple of pieces of fruit or two or more types of vegetables, with some high quality oil. Protein foods include fish, poultry, eggs, nuts and nut butter, seeds, soy products, legumes, and protein powders. If you do well on grains, you can add them into your meals as well. For more information about calcium sources, see the chapters on calcium.

I make a one-week food rotation for 21 meals, which I change from time to time to keep myself interested and to take seasonal availability into account. Here are some tips: Use a pencil and 21 little pieces of paper. With the help of the food family tables, write down a different meal on every piece of paper and then arrange them until you have the week the way you want it. Skip at least one day between foods that are from the same botanical family. Try to plan meals so you don't eat a calcium-rich food with one that contains a calcium antagonist. (More info about this in later chapters). Plan lots of vegetables into your rotation to help combat laziness (like mine) about making vegetables. When your plan is ready, write it onto a single piece of paper that goes on the fridge door and use it to shop, since it's easy to see what needs to be replaced.

If all this sounds unbelievably mysterious and complicated, don't try to figure out seven days worth of meals. Start slowly. Observe your eating habits over a week and then change just *one* thing. If you always eat cereal in the morning, try a power shake with fruit, protein powder, and a tablespoon of hempseed or Udo's oil. Or try fruit with nuts or nut butter for breakfast. Or have leftover salad with fish or chicken. There's no rule that says you always have to eat cereal and toast at breakfast. Eventually, you may work out four to seven different morning meals. Then, if you wish, move on to altering some of your other daily meals. For ideas, see the chapters on *Meal and Snack Ideas.*

Making a food plan does become easier as you familiarize yourself with the ideas in the following chapters on food and start to make a few changes. Give yourself lots of time. The beauty of a food rotation plan is that it's a customized plan you make for yourself, respecting your own likes and dislikes. And you can always change it!

64. TAKE ENZYMES.

Enzymes are incredibly important to the body and are used for many, many vital functions. Without enzymes, you'd be dead.

Your body creates many enzymes but they must respond to numerous demands and stresses. When you maintain high levels of nutrition, you assist them with their work instead of creating more problems for them to handle. Lots of enzymes are used up daily, especially for digestion. Since you produce fewer digestive enzymes as you get older, it's a good idea to do everything you can to add to your supply.

Cooking and commercial food-processing methods kill enzymes. Other culprits that destroy or interfere with enzyme production and digestion are stress, drinking liquids with meals (especially very cold liquids), drugs including caffeine and alcohol, and pollutants in food, water or air. Because stress is so hard on enzymes, it helps to eat meals in a relaxed, pleasant atmosphere. Perhaps this is one of the reasons the French have such low levels of heart problems, despite a diet that is high in animal fats and their fondness for smoking. They know how to enjoy their meals.

If you're used to having your meals while watching violent programs on television, reading the newspaper or experiencing strong negative emotions, try turning off the t.v., putting down the paper and calming down first with deep breathing, a time-out or a short meditation or prayer. Even if you are able to eat calmly for one meal per day, your digestive system—and your whole body—will be happier for it.

You can increase your enzyme supply by eating raw foods, since all raw foods contain their own enzymes. Fruits and vegetables, sea vegetables, alfalfa, fresh herbs, and sprouted grains fall into this category. But if most of your foods to date have been cooked or processed, bring more raw foods *slowly* into your diet. Your body will have to get used to digesting them! Juicing, or grinding up raw fruits and vegetables in a blender or food processor may help.

Another way to increase enzymes that help with digestion is to take enzyme supplements with meals. Look for a broad-spectrum, natural-source digestive enzyme such as Udo's Choice, or Ultra-Zyme by Nu-Life. Broad-spectrum means the enzymes will digest protein, fat (lipids), and carbohydrates. According to David Keith, R.N.C., you need both pancreatic enzymes, which do their work in the small intestine, and plant enzymes, which help digest the food in the stomach. Good quality enzyme supplements are available in natural foods stores.

A second type of enzyme is systemic oral enzymes. These are not purely for digestion but, according to Michael Loes, M.D. and David Steinman, M.A. in *The Aspirin Alternative*, assist in healing chronic and acute pain, as well as inflammatory conditions such as arthritis or sports injuries. They particularly recommend the well-documented Wobenzym N.

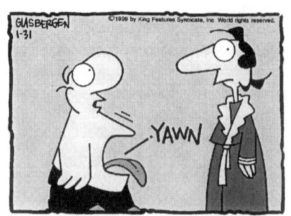

"I've got to stop eating so much.
My stomach was awake all
night digesting my dinner."

65. BE CAREFUL WITH MOLDY AND YEASTY FOODS.

Foods that contain mold and yeast are implicated in numerous health problems including candida (an overgrowth of a yeast that occurs naturally in the body), asthma, arthritis, allergies, tiredness, depression, and fungal infections and growths. If you or your family have a history of any of these conditions, you may want to be careful with fermented foods—soy sauce, vinegar, beer, wine, alcohol, pickles, and olives in brine. Moldy and yeasty foods also include mushrooms, cheeses, peanuts, yeasted breads, dried fruits, and the skins of some fresh fruits, such as apples, pears, and grapes. If you crave these foods or their juices, observe how you react after consuming them—if you don't feel great, try eliminating them for a while and see if there's an improvement. Try peeling your apples and pears.

Rinsing dried fruit with boiling water before eating will remove some mold or yeast. Rinse a whole bag of dried fruit at a time, then store whatever you don't immediately use in a glass jar in the freezer to prevent any further mold or yeast growth. Always remove moldy or black spots from vegetables and don't eat old bananas or other over-ripe fruit. Mold grows long roots which may not be visible, so when removing a dark spot from a fruit or veggie always cut out a large section around the spot.

66. BUY ORGANICALLY-GROWN OR AT LEAST AVOID THE MOST CHEMICALLY-POLLUTED CROPS.

There are five excellent reasons to eat organically-grown foods.

1. *No chemicals.* Organically-grown food is *not* produced with synthetic fertilizers and pesticides, growth regulators, antibiotics, hormones, radiation, and synthetic additives and colorings. Organic growers usually avoid foods created in bio-technology labs as there is a great deal of controversy over the long-term effects of bio-engineered foods on human health, species diversity, and food safety.

2. *More nutrients.* Organically-grown produce consistently shows higher levels of vitamins and minerals than produce from chemical farms.

Most food in North America and other countries practicing monoculture farming is grown in soil that has been overworked for so long there are no nutrients left in it to go into the plants. Chemical fertilizers and pesticides are required to make the same crop grow over and over in the same field.

Foods that are full of chemicals instead of nutrients have little to offer your body. Some foods are so denatured, they don't contain enough nutrients for you to digest and assimilate them. Eating them can give you indigestion and, in the long run, contribute to degenerative conditions.

3. *Better taste.* Organically-grown food tastes much better to me than chemically-grown. Why? It may be because organically-grown foods contain such high levels of nutrients compared to commercially-raised. Perhaps the extra nutrients provide more flavor. Or it may simply be the lack of bitter and unpleasant-tasting chemical residues in the food. Either way, top chefs in the finest establishments know that organic food tastes best, and prefer to use organically-grown ingredients whenever they can.

4. *Sustainable agriculture.* Organic food is grown with sustainable

farming practices. This means the environment is not harmed by the farming methods and crops are interspersed and rotated, so the nutients in the soil are not exhausted.

Commercial, agri-business farming, on the other hand, puts a *huge* amount of pollution into the earth, the air, and your water supply. It is extremely resource-intensive and very hard on the land. Agriculture, according to science writer, Janine Benyus, "is the number one polluting industry" in North America!

5. *Human and animal safety.* Overfarming of cattle is one reason for outbreaks of deadly E. coli in municipal water supplies. Hoof and mouth disease and the consequent destruction of thousands of animals has been linked to commercial farming practices involving the use of dead animals in feed for herbivores.

Organic farms do not rely on chemicals and genetically-altered crops. In contrast to agri-business farms, they do *not* pour hundreds of gallons of chemicals and drugs into our drinking water, polluting the environment for all living creatures and creating dangerous bacterial responses. When you buy organically-grown food, you are supporting your own health *and* the health of the planet.

The organic food category shows continuous annual increases in North America and is growing even faster in Europe, making healthy choices consistently more available to consumers at better prices. There are many ways to purchase organic foods without spending a fortune. Some families buy a share in a Consumer Supported Agriculture farm, visit organic farmers' markets and pick-your-own farms, or belong to an organic food co-op.

Foods to beware of:

Until organic foods become as widely available as agri-business foods, many of us will continue to buy commercially-grown produce. Even so, there are a few items that are so heavily contaminated with pesticides and chemical residues, you should make the extra effort to purchase these organically-grown or don't buy them at all, especially if you have kids.

Children are growing, so they eat a lot more food than adults relative to their size and take in more toxins proportionately. Because their systems are still developing, they are especially vulnerable to the allergenic, carcinogenic, mutagenic, neurotoxic, and hormone-disrupting effects of pesticides and chemical fertilizers and should be protected from them at all costs. Elderly people and those with compromised immunity are also at greater risk, but let's face it, chemically-grown food is hard on everybody.

The conventionally-grown foods to watch out for are: strawberries— strawberries that are not organically-grown have the highest levels of pesticides of any food!—bananas, apples, peaches, green and red peppers, especially from Mexico, canteloupe from Mexico, green beans, celery, pears, apricots, cucumbers, spinach, rice, oats, grapes from Chile, baby food, and soy products. Beware of these items if grown in North America, but be warier of them if imported, since the pesticide use in other countries is even worse! (Pesticides banned here are often sold to other countries.)

Protect yourself with organically-grown versions of these foods.

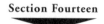

TESTING & DETOXING

67. TESTING FOR SENSITIVITIES.

Caution: Anyone who has extreme allergic responses or comes from a family where there are known allergies requiring medical attention must be tested only by a physician who can provide medical help in case of an anaphylactic reaction during testing. If your regular physician is unable to provide you with the testing option you choose, seek out an M.D. who is a clinical ecologist or specialist in environmental medicine.

Why test for sensitivities, especially if you think you don't react to anything? Testing gives you some important clues about how to support your health. Most of us have recurring themes in our responses to life whether they come in the form of headaches, digestive problems, skin reactions, PMS, depression, aching joints, breathing problems or other reactions. Testing will help you learn what may be causing these responses so you can decide what to do about them before they develop into more serious health problems. You can also use testing to make good choices about products and substances that will be in your body and your life, and to find out which foods work well for you, so you can choose to eat them more often.

What is the difference between an allergy and a sensitivity or intolerance?

An allergy is a medically-recognized condition involving an *unusual* level of sensitivity to an insect bite, a food, or some other substance. Those of us who do not have allergic reactions may still react to many substances, but have more subtle responses, called sensitivities or intolerances. A sensitivity is a signpost, an indication that your body and/or nervous system is struggling with one or more stressors and is signalling you to take action. Sensitivity or intolerance is not currently recognized by many physicians unless they are clinical ecologists or specialists in environmental medicine. Why this is so, only the medical profession can say.

According to medical doctors Stuart Berger and Doris Rapp, testing by traditional scratch or injection methods or by radioimmuno-assay often shows inaccurate results. They suggest these tests may be more useful for the extremely allergic than for people who react more subtly and observe that because many symptoms of sensitivity or intolerance are not disease symptoms, they may be dismissed as mere discomfort or imagination on the part of the sufferer.

Medical doctors specializing in clinical ecology or environmental medicine and naturopaths can provide testing to uncover the underlying causes of sensitivity or intolerance. A non-medical health practitioner or wellness consultant may also provide testing and evaluation to determine what lifestyle or other controllable factors contribute to your state of health. Increasingly, these services receive insurance coverage as the economic value of preventative treatment becomes obvious.

Where to start:

There are several methods of testing for sensitivities and intolerances. These range from medical scratch tests to computer methods to applied kinesiology (muscle testing). Methods vary in cost, effectiveness, and time they require to be performed. Some provide more information than others about where and how the body is affected.

You can cut back significantly on the amount of testing you pay for by using the information in this book to eliminate all known chemical toxins from your home. Since perfumed products, solvents, pesticides, and chemicals burden *everyone's* immune system and cause health problems, your whole family stands to benefit when your house becomes a haven from these pollutants. Instead of chemical toxins, focus your testing on less obvious areas: foods, virus, candida, dental materials, or anything you feel uncertain about.

Testing Methods:

Consumers can choose from a number of options. Charges for these services are usually by the hour. The number of sessions you need for testing and corrective therapy or treatment will depend on the state of your health and how much you're willing to contribute to your own well-being by making necessary lifestyle changes. Some people need only a few initial sessions and then an occasional follow-up appointment during stressful times, whether seasonal, physical or emotional. Seasonal stress could be mold or pollen in spring or fall and chemicals in winter.

• ***Computer biofeedback*** methods include technologies such as Interro machines, Omega AcuBase Technology, and the Quantum Xeroid System. In this type of testing, an electronic probe or sensor is pressed against the skin, usually on the hand, while the computer measures the body's electro-magnetic response to a variety of substances.

• *Advantages:* Many substances can be tested quickly; printouts show which are problem substances and what their "rating" is on a scale that indicates body's tolerance levels. This is a non-invasive method, meaning the client does not touch, ingest or inhale any test substance.

• *Disadvantages:* Surface probe can be uncomfortable with continual pressing against finger; some methods do not show which part of body is most affected by the substance.

• *Corrective Therapy:* Homeopathic remedies, herbs, nutrition, and lifestyle counselling.

• ***Applied kinesiology/sensitivity testing*** involves muscle testing the individual to see where a substance weakens the body. Each muscle group is related to an organ, so muscle weakness indicates which organs or areas of the body are affected by the substance. Individual substances in molecular amounts are generally tested through glass. To locate a practitioner, contact your local Kinesiology Association (see Resource Guide.)

• *Advantages:* This is very much a customized approach. When the full range of muscles is tested, the client's body will clearly show exactly where the problems lie. Even very young children and babies can be tested through a surrogate, usually a parent or caregiver. Because substances are tested through glass and do not enter the body—by mouth, nose (via the odor), or injection—it is a very safe, non-invasive method.

• *Disadvantages:* Testing can be time-consuming however this is balanced out by accuracy of information.

• *Corrective Therapy:* Desensitization by exposure to problem substances during neurolymphatic stimulation. Bumps up immune response, contributing to increased levels of general health over time while targeting specific problem areas. Nutrition and lifestyle counselling.

• ***Provocation/Neutralization*** testing is typically done by a physician. It involves individual testing of molecular amounts by mouth or injection, a waiting period to observe the reaction, followed by an antigen (antidote amount) in the case of a negative reaction.

• *Advantages:* Because individual substances are tested (rather than groups of substances), this is a very specific method compared to the usual medical scratch tests.

• *Disadvantages:* This is an invasive method—the substances are taken directly into the body—which can be very hard on the person being tested. Children, particularly, may find internal responses to substances distressing. The testing is time-consuming.

• *Treatment:* Antigen treatment with shots or drops. May require continuous life-long treatment. There may or may not be associated lifestyle education to help the client eliminate causal factors.

A final note:

Testing to discover sensitivities and intolerances can give you information about your body you might never learn otherwise. Because it's a customized approach, it gives you a clearer picture of what works and what doesn't for you personally, so you have more control over your level of health, as well as awareness about what has gone wrong if you don't feel well. Testing can take much of the guess-work out of health. It is a self-empowering choice.

68. SELF-TESTING ON FOODS.

Warning: Never *self-test if there is a history of severe allergic reaction of any kind in your family. Instead, see a physician or qualified health professional.*

If you do *not* have allergies that result in a medical emergency (anaphylactic shock, asthma attack) you can test yourself on foods in your own home. When you react to familiar foods, whether you know you're reacting or not, your system has to work hard to process them and maintain homeostasis. Even if you think you don't have sensitivities, the results of food testing may surprise you!

The first step to take before the testing can begin is to clear your house of all chemicals, plastics, perfumes, and other sources of toxins (see the final chapter: *Top Ten,* for quick reference). This will give you more accurate results. If you test yourself in a house full of chemicals, you won't know whether the results you get are from the food being tested or your home environment.

When clearing out chemicals, be sure to include fabric softeners and scented detergents. Your clothes should be washed with an unscented product and no fabric softener. Wear cotton and natural fiber clothing (including underwear) during the testing period, not synthetics.

Use high quality filtered or distilled water for drinking and brushing teeth, since non-filtered water can be a source of many chemical residues. Because potting soil is a source of mold, put potted plants outside or confine them to an infrequently-used room during the testing period (about a week).

Once your home environment is as toxin-free as possible, you can start testing.

Five-Day Food Elimination Testing to Uncover Sensitivities:

Choose the food to be tested. If you're not sure what to start with, see the list of top allergenic foods at the end of this chapter, and pick one of them. This food must be avoided *completely* for five days. If the item being tested comes in many forms, every form of that food must be eliminated from the diet. For example, if milk is the test food, do not eat *any* dairy product (cheese, butter, ice cream, yogurt, etc.) or any product containing dairy (cheese-coated popcorn, milk chocolate, nachos, etc.) If wheat is being tested, in addition to avoiding the obvious foods like bread and pastries, read labels carefully to ensure there is no unsuspected wheat in items like soups, sauces or snack foods (see chapter 83 on *Flour products & cereal grains* for help). If testing caffeine, be sure to avoid chocolate, hot chocolate, soft drinks, black tea and green tea.

Eating or inhaling molecular amounts of a substance can affect a sensitive individual, just as the smell of cigarette smoke in the air affects non-smokers or a pinch of disliked spice can be tasted in a recipe despite being the smallest ingredient. When testing, even tiny amounts of the test food will skew the results, so err on the side of caution. If you're avoiding caffeine, don't go and inhale over the coffee percolator, since this will actually expose you to quite a lot of airborne caffeine molecules. If avoiding wheat, you may be affected by the smell of bread toasting or the fresh-baked odors in a bakery, so don't go pastry shopping for someone else. It might sound extreme but, what the heck, it's only for a week!

How the test works:

During the five days of avoidance, your body clears out residues of the selected food. At the end of five days, you reintroduce the test food to discover your body's true reaction to it, for better or worse! Your reaction when the food is brought back will show whether or not you have an intolerance to it, and how you're affected by the food.

During the five days of avoidance, you may experience cravings and/or withdrawal symptoms. They might be physical ones like headaches, fatigue, itchiness, and flu-like symptoms, or mental and emotional ones like confusion, forgetting, depression or tearfulness. They will pass. Keep away from the test food at all costs!

Intense craving is a sign of sensitivity or intolerance to a food. It's normal to crave the food you react to worst, in order to continue the masking effect.

When you're sensitive to a food and you keep eating it, your body copes by masking its true reaction. Masking uses up huge amounts of nutrients and enzymes that would otherwise go towards nourishing and healing your body. To maintain the masking effect, you have to eat the problem food at regular intervals. If you wait too long for a "dose" of the food, the masking effect begins to wear off and you feel uncomfortable. As your discomfort increases, you find yourself craving the substance. This is similar to what is experienced by the chronic smoker, drinker or drug addict.

After five days, you can eat the restricted food again. But be careful! The reason you're eating it this time is to find out your body's *true* reaction to the food. That reaction may not be pleasant, so don't eat a big portion. In fact, you may want to eat just *one* bite—that can be plenty—then wait and see what happens. For an even more cautious approach to reintroducing the food, see below.

Possible reactions will range in type and severity, and can be physical or emotional, since many foods act as neurotoxins, or both. You might experience coughing, sneezing, stomach ache, headache, intestinal gas, tiredness, feeling "funny", runny nose or eyes, itchy skin, wobbly knees or shaking legs, glassy eyes, sudden anger or irritation, depression, weepiness, disorientation, feeling spaced out or more forgetful than usual or uncoordinated and clumsy.

Or you could feel okay initially and then have a delayed reaction. The food has to process all the way through the digestive system before it is eliminated and your reaction to it might occur at any point in this process. You need to be able to pay attention to yourself over a period of several hours, checking to see if something unusual is occuring. This might be easier on a weekend than a work day.

According to Dr. Doris Rapp, delayed reactions include ear and bowel problems, tight joints and, in children, bedwetting. You may also develop skin irritation or a headache. If I eat dairy, I react to it the *following* day, by sneezing and coughing up mucus.

When you're quite sensitive to a food, even a molecular amount can affect you. To be sure you don't suffer any really uncomfortable reactions, try the following:

1. After the five days are up and you want to try the test food again, first, *sniff* the food. Wait. If no reaction, proceed to 2.

Note: Choose as pure a version of the food as possible. For example, use plain milk or yogurt when testing dairy. If you test with flavored yogurt or milk, you won't know whether you're reacting to the fruit, sugar or other ingredient, or to the dairy. Similarly, test wheat with plain pasta or cream of wheat cereal rather than bread, which contains yeast and other ingredients.

2. Rub a little of the food on your skin, or hold some against your abdomen, near the navel. Remember, the body is an integrated system, which transmits messages from one location to all parts of itself. As any quantum physicist can tell you, anything that enters your energy field can have an effect on you. So if the food is going to make you cough, just holding it against your stomach may be enough to cause the coughing to start, depending on how sensitive you are to the food.

Again, wait and watch. If you have a reaction, remove the food or wash off immediately. If no reaction, proceed to:

3. Put a little of the food to your lips, but do not eat it. If no reaction, proceed to:

4. Take a small bite of the food and simply hold it in your mouth without eating it. If you react, spit it out immediately. If no reaction, proceed to:

5. Eat one small bite of the food. Wait and observe, noting reactions. Some will be instantaneous, others will take as long as six to eight hours to show up.

If all these trials are passed successfully with no reaction, congratulations! It's not *that* food which is the problem. There are lots to try. In general, however, the top allergenic foods are the ones to check first—dairy, wheat, corn, sugar, caffeine and chocolate, oranges, apples, peanuts, yeast, pork, and foods with additives and colors.

As you can see, this process can take a bit of time and effort. But it's free!

69. WHAT HAPPENS WHEN YOUR BODY CLEARS OUT TOXINS? ABOUT DETOXING.

When you cut out foods that don't agree with you and products made with powerful chemicals, an odd thing can happen. Before you feel better, you might feel worse! You could find you're extremely tired, your nose runs, or you feel nauseous or headachy. You might even think you're coming down with a cold. There can be emotional symptoms too: sadness, anger, irritability. These symptoms could last several hours or a few days!

What's really happening? Are you sick? Are you going crazy? No, you're *detoxing.*

When you stop a problem food or chemical or other toxin, you "unmask" your body's real symptoms. Now the ugly truth comes out. You may also find yourself detoxing after a session of massage therapy, acupuncture, reflexology or other type of body work, as toxins are released from cells and exit the body. Don't worry! Your symptoms, uncomfortable as they are, will pass.

Detoxification is a strange experience. You're not sick, but you don't exactly feel well, either. I have been through detoxes that included both physical and emotional reactions: aches and pains, soreness, headache, depression, lethargy, and feeling vulnerable and moody. Fortunately this only lasts for a day or two. Sometimes it's not the day after I stop a problem substance that I feel bad, it's the day *after* the day after!

Will you detox the same way as me? Not necessarily. Lots of people detox without any particular discomfort. Still, it's just as well to be prepared, physically and emotionally. When there are negative emotional reactions, I find it helps to remind myself they are only temporary results of the detox.

If you find out you're like me and have tiring detoxes, plan accordingly. Don't take a treatment or plan a major change in your eating or living habits if you're going through a stressful time, it's holiday season, or you're embarking on a tour of the vineyards of France. Choose a later date to detox.

Sometimes detoxing is not uncomfortable, but takes time. One woman had eczema all over her body. She discovered she was very sensitive to chemicals, tap water, some foods, and to her prescription cortisone cream. After she got the toxins out of her home, water supply, and diet, her eczema began to disappear. The clearing of her skin condition began at her feet and moved slowly upward to her head, over a period of weeks. The very last places to become eczema-free were the areas of her face where she'd used the cortisone cream! Although her detox was not uncomfortable, it did require considerable patience while her body went through its healing process.

Once you've cleaned up your home environment and diet, here are some techniques to help your body clear out toxins, especially chemical toxins. Both Udo Erasmus, Ph.D., and Andrew Weil, M.D., recommend sweating in a sauna or steam bath to help release toxins from the cells. Bring along some good quality drinking water to help yourself remain hydrated while sweating.

Another helpful method is to massage or tap lymphatic areas. Lymphatic fluid, as part of the immune system, helps to clear toxins from the body. But the lymph has one obstacle. While your circulation has your heart to keep it moving, the lymph has no such means of locomotion.

That's where you come in. You can help your lymph to move, so it moves toxins out of your body, by having a lymph massage or massaging lymphatic areas yourself. Try massaging in small circles or tap with your fingertips all around the chest area, hips, thighs, neck, and upper arms. Always massage in the direction of your heart. Exercise helps the lymph to move, particularly jumping on a trampoline or mini-trampoline. Finish off with a baking soda, sea salt or epsom salt bath to draw even more chemical toxins out of your system. Or lie down on a slant with your feet higher than your head for fifteen minutes or so. If you can manage a headstand, that's good too. This inverted posture will send your lymph flowing in a different direction than usual, stimulate your circulation, and help food move through your intestines.

Some foods help to bind chemicals and excrete them. These include sea vegetables (seaweeds), green leafy vegetables, and cruciferous vegetables such as broccoli. Eat them regularly to help your body detoxify chemicals you encounter daily.

MEAL & SNACK IDEAS

70. MEAL IDEAS YOU MAY NOT HAVE CONSIDERED. BREAKFAST.

As a North American, I went along with the philosophy that I was one of a continent of independent thinkers moving fearlessly in the direction of progress. Until someone told me I could eat something other than cereal or toast for breakfast. That's when I found out how conservative I really was! (If you want to know what people really *believe* in, try getting them to change their eating habits.) No cereal?! No toast?! As Samuel Goldwyn said, "In two words, im possible!"

After I recovered from the shock of discovering familiar meal ideas were not laws of nature but cultural habits, I began experimenting. What worked well for my body? What didn't?

Cereal and toast, because they are grain-based, didn't work all that well for me on a daily basis. In fact, when I paid attention to my body's messages, I realized too much of these foods made me tired and hungry and gave me indigestion. Once I stopped eating grains in the morning every day, I no longer needed coffee or chocolate to keep me awake.

Some nutrition experts recommend eating only fruit for breakfast. Since fruit is natural sugars, water, and fiber with some vitamins and minerals, it's wonderful for cleansing the system or as *part* of a meal. But by itself, it can unbalance the blood sugar. If you're still hungry or feel spaced out an hour after you eat it, fruit alone isn't enough. You need protein and fat for a balanced meal and to feel satisfied.

Nuts and nut butter contain protein and fat. They can be added to your breakfast fruit. When you're in a rush, a piece of fruit and a handful of nuts is a fast, easy meal you can carry with you. If you tolerate dairy foods, try fruit and yogurt or cheese for breakfast. Creamy goat cheese is delicious on pears or apples.

Another option is to make a breakfast shake. Buy protein powder made from organically grown soy or rice (particularly if you're dairy-sensitive). Put a couple of tablespoons of it into a cup of filtered water in the blender. Add a banana or other piece of fruit and some food-based nutrient powder like The Missing Link, Udo's Choice Wholesome Fast Food Blend, or Greens +. Whiz that into a thick shake and pour into a glass. Then stir in a tablespoon of high quality oil rich in essential fatty acids (EFA's). Choose hempseed oil or Udo's Oil Blend.

If you prefer, you can blend in a tablespoon of nut butter instead of oil, although you won't get the same EFA benefits. Macadamia, almond, cashew or tahini are good choices. Bear in mind that almond and cashew butter and soy protein powder all contain calcium antagonists, so they are best used together (the Fast Food Blend contains soy). If you use rice protein powder and macadamia butter or tahini, there are no calcium antagonists.

You can still eat soy, almond, and cashew. Just rotate them through the week with other foods. The worst thing you can do is to eat *exactly* the same thing for breakfast or any other meal, every day for the rest of your life. Your body thrives on variety and gets more nutrients when you vary your foods.

Speaking of variety, who says you have to eat any particular type of food in the morning? We have a friend who sometimes eats meat or chicken with salad or veggies for breakfast. She always has good energy and concentration for her work when she eats this way. Like me, she finds grains put her to sleep.

What if you love cereal and tolerate grains well? Eat a variety and select whole grains over flour products. (For more information, see chapter on *Achieving grain variety*.) Granola and energy or power bars are probably not the best choice at breakfast as they tend to have a high sugar content.

For hot cereal, try something other than oatmeal or cream of wheat to prevent your body from developing a reaction to these familiar grains. Cook up some 90-second quinoa (made by Ancient Harvest), or, if you have time, a pot of millet. Millet cooked with bananas and raisins or dates is delicious. To save time, cook a big batch of hot cereal such as plain millet, quinoa or sweet rice and freeze in individual portions. Then heat with fresh or dried fruit at breakfast time. These cereals do not require milk unless you prefer them with it. Try soy, rice or almond beverages. To sweeten hot cereals, use a little maple syrup or honey, or cook them with raisins or dates. Cold cereals such as spelt, kamut or millet, puffed or in flakes, are another possibility. Eaten with soy or almond beverage, they will provide complete protein.

Fond of eggs and toast or a big pancake breakfast? Choose the healthiest possible versions of these meals. Buy free-range eggs, organic spelt or kamut bread, organic butter, and fruit spread sweetened with fruit juice (called jam when it's sweetened with sugar.) Use sea salt and drink organically-grown coffee or decaf, if you're a coffee-lover. Make pancakes with oat, buckwheat or spelt flour and spread them with organic butter and maple syrup or nut butter and fruit spread.

Why go to the trouble of buying all this organic food, and alternatives to regular bread and pancakes? Because you will *significantly* reduce the quantity of pesticides, preservatives, artificial colors, and drug and hormone residues you would ingest from conventional food products. At the same time, you will significantly increase your available nutrients. Free-range eggs, for example, are rich in the essential fatty acids vital to your body's ability to function correctly. Eggs from chickens who live their whole lives in boxes, on the other hand, are nutrient-poor and lack essential fatty acids. While it's a good idea to vary the foods you eat at breakfast, it may be less important to change the *type* of food you eat than to upgrade its quality.

71. LUNCH AND DINNER.

Because grains make me tired, I stopped eating sandwiches or pasta at lunch and tried eating protein and veggies instead. The results? Significantly more energy that lasted all afternoon and no more of that 4 p.m.

sag that made me want to nap or drink coffee. The most amazing part is how much my food cravings diminished. When I ate grains at lunch, because of the way they affected my blood sugar, I would often want to eat again a couple of hours later. But once I switched to protein and vegetables, my body was able to run on that fuel for hours, without feeling hungry.

You may feel perfectly well and energized on grains. If so, wonderful! But if you've experienced symptoms like mine or you know you react poorly to grains, experiment with not eating them and see what happens. Violent cravings for grain products when you go off them can indicate an intolerance. You will tend to be addictively attracted to the food that's hardest on you. (See chapters on *testing for sensitivities.*)

So, for lunch, protein and veggies can mean less fatigue, more and longer lasting energy over the afternoon, and better ability to concentrate at work, school or anything you do that requires focus and attention. You don't need a lot of protein, nor does it have to be from an animal source. In fact, the amount of fat usually attached to animal protein can put you to sleep as fast as a reaction to grains. In his book, *10 Natural Remedies That Can Save Your Life*, James Balch, M.D., suggests that if you happen to eat a high-fat meal, some of the negative effects can be moderated by taking vitamins C and E with the food or as soon as possible afterwards. Digestive enzymes help, too. Carry some with you when eating away from home.

At dinner, unless you have evening classes or meetings, you can play around a bit more with what you're going to eat. If you can relax and don't have to work in a focussed way after dinner, this is the best time of day to eat grain carbohydrates. Try changing the elements of your usual dinner to take any strain off your immune system.

For example, if you like pasta, buy some whole grain noodles made from rice, spelt, kamut, buckwheat or quinoa, and eat them with your favorite sauce. If you always eat tomato sauce, try cooking other vegetables to blend with olive oil as a substitute sauce. If you use prepackaged, chemically-preserved parmesan out of a can or bottle on your sauce, give yourself a treat. Go to a cheese shop and ask for pecorino romano—this is the original cheese for grating onto pasta, made from sheep's milk. It's delicious. You can grate it yourself by hand or in the food processor, then store the leftover in a jar in the freezer.

If you're a meat and potatoes person and you always eat butter on your spuds, buy organic butter and organic milk or sour cream for mashed potatoes. This will ensure you do not eat the antibiotics and growth hormones in regular dairy. Or, if you want to try going dairy-free, slather your potatoes with olive oil. Add garlic, if you like it, for a natural immune boost and delicious flavor.

Switch from iodized table salt to natural sea salt. Iodized salt may contain sugar and chemicals or metals (aluminum, silicates) to keep it from sticking together. To keep moisture out of my sea salt, I store it in a jar with a hard plastic lid (salt corrodes metal lids). I've also seen attractive wooden boxes for sea salt. Or put your sea salt into a salt shaker with grains of rice to absorb any moisture and allow the salt to run freely. If you need iodine, eat dulse, wakame, kelp or other seaweeds instead of iodized salt.

Seaweeds, also called sea vegetables, are a good source of nutrients. You can buy powdered seaweeds to sprinkle over salads, popcorn or any food for a zing of oceany taste. If you're not fond of that flavor, hide the seaweed in stews, sauces or casseroles. Most seaweeds provide calcium and a mixture of other minerals and vitamins.

Cook your foods in the healthiest possible way. Foods fried in fat—especially lard, margarine, and processed vegetable oil—or deep fried are tremendously hard on your body. Frying chemically changes fat molecules and creates lots of free radicals associated with cancer and other diseases. When you see the oil in your pan smoking, it has gone toxic.

Instead of frying in fat or oil, put some water in the pan first, then some high quality oil that will survive heating, such as olive oil. The water keeps the oil from overheating, since the temperature can only go up to boiling temp instead of the extreme highs of fat frying, so the oil is less likely to change into a toxin.

Or just leave out the oil and cook in water. You can add the oil after the food is cooked. Never use lard, margarine or hydrogenated fats. If you need a hardened fat, organic butter is the best choice. People have been eating it for thousands of years, whereas margarine has only been around since the 1950's. *The Power of Superfoods* author, Sam Graci, among others, cautions against margarine, warning it may be treated with petrochemical solvents. Lard is either manufactured from altered oils, or, if it's from animal fat, it will contain high levels of pesticides and other toxins.

When baking, use baking paper as chefs do, instead of greasing the pan or cookie sheet. Baking the "grease" overheats it and makes it toxic. Baking paper is easy to use and keeps your pans cleaner so you have less washing-up to do afterwards.

Instead of frying meat, fish and chicken, bake, broil or grill at a temperature that will not blacken them. The charred part of any food is considered carcinogenic. If you burn your toast or your barbecued food, scrape or cut off the black part.

Try to include a leafy green vegetable with as many meals as possible for calcium and antioxidants. This could be lettuce, salad greens, parsley, alfalfa sprouts, collard greens, asparagus, broccoli, dandelion greens, cabbage or well-cooked kale or chard.

Dinner at our house is fairly plain—vegetables and a protein, occasionally a whole grain or whole grain pasta with vegetables. If you love to cook and crave more elaborate yet health-oriented recipes, explore vegetarian cookbooks. There are some fabulous recipes in Deborah Madison's *Vegetarian Cooking for Everyone*, and in *Linda McCartney on Tour—Over 200 Meat-free Recipes from Around the World*. These books emphasize fresh, natural ingredients. They tell you how to make whole grain dishes and baked goods, plan meals (to which you can simply add a meat course if you are a meat-eater), and provide delectable ways to get more veggies into your life. There are even sugar-free desserts!

Another terrific book is Lisa Turner's *Meals that Heal*, which provides delicious, uncomplicated recipes full of antioxidants and phytochemicals—health-giving, disease-resisting substances that occur naturally in various foods.

72. SNACK IDEAS.

• Cut fruit and vegetables into bite-sized pieces and store in fridge for quick snacks. Kids love this!

• Rice cakes with nut butter, soy or rice cheese-substitutes or goat cheese. Mini rice cakes are good cracker substitutes or try whole grain crackers.

• Unsulphured dried fruit and/or uncoated nuts. Stay away from "dry-roasted" and flavored nuts in the grocery store. They are usually coated with irradiated spices, sugar, flour, and chemical preservatives.

• Calcium-rich trail mix of nuts, sunflower seeds, pumpkin seeds, unsweetened carob chips which are naturally sweet, and raisins or other dried fruit—apricots, dates, chopped figs. Avoid peanuts, which may carry aflatoxin, a fungal carcinogen.

• Fruit "leathers" or roll-ups sweetened with fruit juice, not sugar. Kettle Valley Dried Fruit Co. makes a delicious organic fruit bar.

• Rice-based puddings in individual serving sizes, at natural foods stores and some grocers.

• Carob 'hot chocolate', made with unsweetened carob powder and soy, rice or nut beverage. If desired, sweeten with honey.

• Hot chocolate made with organic chocolate powder and soy, rice or nut beverage, and honey. Or try it with Edenblend rice/soy beverage, a rich-tasting drink, and no sweetener.

• Individual soymilks in various flavors, from natural foods stores and some grocers.

• Wheat-free muffins made with spelt, oat or kamut flour. Add raisins, berries, nuts or carob chips.

• Organic popcorn or organic corn chips. For extra nutrients and flavor, sprinkle popcorn with Udo's or hempseed oil, kelp powder, and an herb of your choice, such as tarragon or basil. Salt with sea salt or a few squirts of organic soy sauce.

• Whole grain cookies sweetened with fruit juice, barley malt or rice syrup.

• Honey-sweetened nut & seed bars.

Note: If you are a sweet-lover who can polish off most of a bag of cookies as a snack, consider eating fruit or dried fruit as your sweet instead. Even if you binge on these items, they contain *considerably* more nutrients than cookies and other baked sweets and, because they are full of fiber, you will eliminate them fairly rapidly. Baked products, on the other hand, tend to block up your intestines (unless you have a gluten allergy, in which case, they may give you diarrhea.) Also, if you can eat large amounts of sweets without feeling satisfied, see chapters on: *If you crave sweets, don't blame yourself. Blame your chemistry.* and *Sugar and blood sugar. What's the difference?*

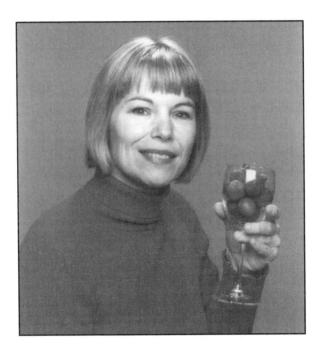

Protein, Fats & Oils

73. PROTEIN.

For many years in our culture, animal protein has been the centerpiece of a meal: a large serving of red meat with potatoes and a small amount of vegetable on the side. Many restaurants still cater to this concept of eating, although more and more people have switched to eating fish and chicken instead of red meat. Even with this change, protein from the animal world is the main ingredient.

The healthier choice is to eat the meat, chicken or fish like a condiment, with a small serving added to a much larger amount of vegetables. This is closer to the traditional diet of long-lived, healthy peoples in various parts of the world.

Do you tend to eat one big dose of protein per day, like a big steak or chicken breast at lunch or dinner, while the rest of the day you consume mostly carbohydrates—bakery products, fruit, cereal, pop, and chips? Try spreading your protein out over the day, so you eat moderate amounts at every meal and snack. When I made this change, I experienced an increase in my energy level, more balanced emotions, and improved concentration.

It's a good idea to vary the types of protein you eat during a day. Unless you're vegetarian, have a little animal protein (chicken, fish, eggs) at one meal—but not too much, since heavy meat meals pass through the intestines very slowly. Diverticulitis, colon cancer, and other health problems related to the digestive organs may be related to this slow transit time. Consuming lots of fresh, leafy vegetables with the meat, fish or chicken will help move it along quickly. At your other meals, eat some protein from plant sources: nuts, beans, seeds, soy, and vegetables (although veggies by themselves are quite low in protein). This way, you'll get a whole range of amino acids and nutrients and your body won't miss out on any of them.

Plant-source proteins are sometimes called "incomplete" because they contain varying amounts of amino acids, so you have to mix them together for complete protein. The idea with these incomplete proteins is to mix *any* legume, nut, seed or protein powder with any grain or mixture of vegetables. This will give you all the amino acids. Foodwise, it looks like this: beans and rice, whole-grain bread and nut butter, salad with sunflower seeds or walnuts, hummus with pita bread, and so on. Any good, recent vegetarian cookbook will contain lots of delicious recipes providing complete protein.

Judge your protein needs according to your physical requirements. People who are young or very active need more protein—for growth and muscle—than people who are sedentary or elderly. Also, people who are sugar-sensitive or who have mercury amalgam fillings may require a little extra protein daily and definitely need protein regularly throughout the day in order to feel well.

One caveat about fish: ocean fish are generally safer than those caught in fresh water, unless you know the lake is clear of industrial pollutants or agricultural run-off. Fish caught in the Great Lakes are *highly* contaminated with pesticides and chemical residues.

Women of child-bearing age—from puberty onwards—should be especially careful as these toxins accumulate in body fat and are passed on to your fetus. If you're pregnant, avoid Great Lakes fish *completely*. Studies have shown that children of mothers who eat Great Lakes fish before and during their pregnancies can have serious neurological impairment and behavior problems.

Milk and meat are two other areas of concern. Domestic livestock are often fed on pesticide-treated crops and the remains of other animals, and may contain bovine growth hormone, antibiotics, and infectious prion proteins causing BSE (mad cow disease). Bovine IGF-I is considered a key element in the growth of breast cancer. For safety, choose organic milk and meat from livestock grown on plant foods without drugs.

Always eat a little oil with your protein, as this helps it digest and assimilate. Nature arranges for this to a certain extent by making sure most protein foods contain some fat, however, if you are eating a protein powder, non-fatty fish (most small, white ocean fish are low in fat) without the skin or plant protein such as legumes, you may need to supplement the meal with some high-quality oil.

74. EAT ONLY THE BEST OILS.

Can a book promoting health have anything good to say about fat? Absolutely! Like water, fat is a vital nutrient used in an extraordinary number of physical processes which include helping to regulate heartbeat, ensuring growth to maturity, and digesting protein. According to Udo Erasmus, our brains are 60% fat and need appropriate dietary fats to function. Fats are necessary to immune function. In fact, if you ate no fat, you'd die of a deficiency-related disease!

If fat is something you can't live without, why do you always hear how bad it is for you? Three reasons:

1) *Some* fat is good. North Americans typically eat too much fat.

2) The fats North Americans typically eat too much of are the wrong kind—cooked fats. Heating changes the fat molecule, turning it into a toxin instead of a nutrient. Deep-fat frying is the worst.

3) Most of the vegetable oils and margarines chosen as alternatives to butter are overheated and processed with chemicals. This turns them into toxins. *The harmful effects on the body that are blamed on fats and oils are mostly caused by the chemicals, heat, and destructive processing used to manufacture oils.*

The best oils are uncooked, correctly processed, stored in dark glass bottles and taste fresh and strong, not bland and rancid. They include extra virgin olive oil, hemp oil, and Udo's Choice Oil Blend.

To make sure you are getting the best possible nutrients out of the fat in your diet, you need to do three things:

1) Reduce or eliminate cooked, deep-fried, refined, and hydrogenated fats and oils.

2) Keep animal fats to a minimum since chemical toxins in their feed and water store in the animals' fat cells (just like us!).

3) Focus on eating EFA-rich oils (see chapter on EFAs) and unrefined oils such as extra virgin olive oil as your sources of fat.

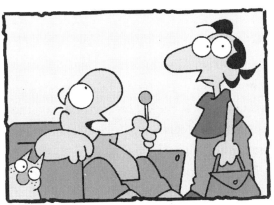

"For dinner I had two beers and
a whole bag of lollipops—
zero grams of fat!"

75. FATS AND OILS: WHICH IS BETTER? REFINED OR LESS POLISHED BUT MORE SINCERE?

Virtually all oils that you find on your supermarket shelf are refined. Extra virgin olive oil is the exception—basically you just get what's been squished out of the olive. Other oils aren't quite so simple.

Extra virgin olive oil keeps well at room temperature without going rancid, particularly if it's in a dark glass bottle. Seed-based or vegetable oils, on the other hand, have three major enemies: light, heat, and oxygen. Any of these three can ruin the oil fairly quickly. To defeat the effects of light, heat, and air, the process used to bring oils from their original seed to the clear plastic bottles you see on the grocer's shelves involves many toxic steps.

Cooking: Seeds are cooked up to two hours before pressing to make the pressing easier. This cracks the seeds and exposes them to air, turning the oil rancid.

Extraction: The oil is extracted from the seedcake mechanically, creating tremendous heat, or with the use of solvents which involves petrochemicals. (Hmm, why buy vegetable oil when you can just pour motor oil on your food?)

Degumming: My favorite part of the processing. Removes fiber, lecithin (important for brain function), iron, calcium, magnesium, copper, and chlorophyll from the oil. Now all the nutrients are gone.

Refining: During the refining process, free fatty acids are removed from the oil by mixing it with sodium hydroxide (also known as drain cleaner), followed by agitation and separation.

Bleaching: Bleaching removes the pigments chlorophyll and beta-carotene from the oil. (You wouldn't think there'd be anything good left in it by now, would you?) Other steps in this process include the use of very high temperatures, resulting in unsafe molecular changes in the oil.

Deodorizing: Because of exposure to heat and air during processing, the oil is now rancid. The rancid taste is burned off—deodorized—using extremely high temperatures. This creates mutagenic fats and the formation of substantial quantities of altered fat molecules.

Now the oil goes into a clear plastic bottle, where, if any nutritious elements have survived, they're killed off by exposure to light. By the time you buy the oil, it's basically toxic waste in a bottle.

When oil is exposed to light, oxygen or heat, as it is when it's refined, changes to its molecular structure occur. Usually, the shape of the molecule changes, making the fat stickier and slower, more likely to clog arteries. Or, the molecules will fit into a cell receptor site but because of the molecular changes will not be able to perform the job required for that cell. Since the site is now occupied, healthy oil molecules can't get in there to do the job properly and the cell suffers. If this only involved one cell in your body, it wouldn't matter, but in eating altered (cooked, rancid, and refined) fats and oils, many, many of your cells are affected, leading to degenerative health and serious disease conditions.

That extra virgin olive oil looks pretty good now, doesn't it?

76. FOCUS ON ESSENTIAL FATTY ACIDS.

Why are essential fatty acids *essential?* Because your body can't manufacture them. The only other place to get them is from the foods you eat and that makes them essential nutrients. Essential to your health, that is. The importance of consuming sufficient amounts of healthy fats and oils on a daily basis cannot be overemphasized. Without them, you turn into a prune—all dried up and wrinkly. Your brain won't work right, either.

One of the components of a healthy fat or oil is the amount of essential fatty acid it contains. There are two "essential" fatty acids (EFAs) our bodies need, not just for health, but *for survival.* These EFAs go by more than one name:
1. W3 essential fatty acid—also known as Alpha-linolenic acid or Omega 3 fatty acid.
2. W6 essential fatty acid—also known as Linoleic acid or Omega 6 fatty acid. The ideal ratio of these EFAs in the diet is 2:1, W3:W6.

Some functions of essential fatty acids:
• EFAs are crucial to the development of the brain in children and to the functioning of the brain in both children and adults.
• EFAs are incorporated into the membrane of every cell in the body. Cells join together to form tissue and tissue joins together to form organs. It follows that membrane health is critical to cell, tissue, and organ health.
• EFAs attract oxygen. Oxygen repels viruses, fungi, bacteria, and other problem organisms from our cells.
• EFAs speed up recovery of muscles from fatigue after heavy exercise whether it's working out in the gym or shovelling snow.
• EFAs contribute substantially to smooth skin, speed of healing, feelings of calmness, and growth rate (maturation of young bodies and youthfulness of older ones).

- EFAs protect you from pesticides.
- EFAs help you lose weight by increasing metabolic rate.

Some symptoms of EFA deficiency:
- Failure to thrive and/or slow growth rate.
- Learning disabilities—can result from mother's deficiency during pregnancy.
- High blood pressure, low metabolic rate.
- Dry skin—the skin is the least important organ and will be deprived of EFAs in favor of internal organs.
- Susceptibility to infection and poor ability to heal.
- Arthritis-like symptoms.
- Heart and/or circulation problems.

Oils high in essential fatty acids:
- Hemp oil: has a 1:3 ratio of W3 and W6
- Udo's Choice Oil Blend: has an optimal 2:1 ratio
- Unrefined safflower oil: has the highest levels of W6
- Unrefined sunflower oil has high W6 levels.

Since North Americans eat a lot of processed food, we tend to lack W3s more than W6s. (Omega 3s perish easily.) Don't cook with the oils listed above—especially don't *fry* with them—since high temperatures destroy EFAs and create toxins.

Focus on getting EFA-rich oils into your diet and reducing or eliminating toxic, rancid, and refined oils, rather than worrying about words like polyunsaturated, monounsaturated, saturated or hydrogenated. These words are tossed around by advertisers, with little regard for your health.

You don't want to eat anything hydrogenated, like hard, processed fats, if you're going to be healthy and your saturated fats, like animal fats, should be kept low. But even a polyunsaturated oil can be trouble unless it's been manufactured correctly, *without* heat, light, air, solvent, and bleach. Good, top-quality EFA-rich oils, like the ones listed above, contain polyunsaturates. Extra virgin olive oil contains monounsaturates and is low in EFAs, so you can cook (gently) with it.

Eggs are another source of essential fatty acids. But only if they are from chickens allowed to range freely, who absorb nutrients allowing them to produce EFA-rich eggs. Free-range eggs are also lower in cholesterol than eggs from box-raised chickens. Don't break the yolk when you cook your eggs as this harms the EFA molecules. You can also get some EFA benefits from Nutiva Shelled Hempseeds and Nutra Sprout™ sprouts.*

Essential fatty acids are so necessary to human health, Udo Erasmus (who wrote *the* book on fats and oils) emphasizes that while it's important to get the bad fats *out* of your diet, you absolutely *must* get the good oils *in*. A diet too low in fat is literally the kiss of death. And since you have to eat fats (or die), you might as well eat the oils that give you the essential fatty acids your body will thrive on. Three to four tablespoons per day of EFA-rich oils—balanced for W3s and W6s—can make a huge positive difference in your physical, mental, and emotional well-being, not to mention your skin quality!

*Certified organic omega-rich Nutra Sprout™ sprouts contain omega 3's.
www.canadianorganicsprouts.com

VEGGIES

77. IS IT BETTER TO BE VEGETARIAN?

First of all, what is vegetarianism? Vegetarians don't eat anything with eyes (except potatoes). No fish, meat, chicken or other birds. Some vegetarians do not eat eggs and some avoid even dairy products.

Is it a better way to eat? Vegetarians would answer yes to this question with excellent reason. Statistics show that vegetarians have lower rates of heart disease, high blood pressure, cancer, and diabetes. And they tend to be less fat than other groups. No one can argue with vegetarians' moral and environmental reasons for eating as they do: fishing and livestock farming need to be conducted more humanely than they are now, and growing plant foods uses up fewer of the earth's resources than animal husbandry by a whopping percentage.

Having said all that, not everyone can be vegetarian. Some bodies simply do not seem to be able to absorb enough protein from vegetable sources. Annemarie Colbin observes that, "vegetarianism works best when accompanied by a deeply felt spiritual commitment", rather than by forcing yourself to eat a vegetarian diet whether or not it makes you feel well. In *Eat Right 4 Your Type*, Peter D'Adamo, N.D., indicates that people with type O and type B blood need animal protein, and only people with type A blood can be true vegetarians. Michael Klaper, M.D., however, is not convinced D'Adamo's theories are correct and thinks people differ in their needs for types of food without being categorized by blood type. Dr. Hal Huggins believes people who have metal in their mouths (fillings, posts, bridgework) must eat animal protein to absorb sufficient amounts of amino acids.

Ultimately, the choice is yours. The determining factor is how you feel. If you feel well physically, mentally, emotionally, and spiritually as a vegetarian, great! Go with it. But if you need a few animal foods in your diet, go with that. The key is balance.

You need to eat enough plant protein on a vegetarian diet or you may feel spaced-out and constantly crave sweets. On the other hand, if you eat huge amounts of animal protein, you can also crave sweets. This second eating pattern of lots of animal protein and fat with anti-nutrient white flour and sugar is one of the causes underlying several "diseases of civilization".

If you are interested in vegetarianism, do some research before beginning. Contact your local vegetarian association. Borrow vegetarian cookbooks from the library and find out how foods are put together to provide enough amino acids and other nutrients. Make sure you get complete protein by combining different plant foods at every meal. Be aware that vegetarians can run short on vitamin B-12, so plan good sources into your diet (this deficiency forms over two or three years so don't wait for it to happen. It can result in a very serious form of anemia that is difficult to reverse.) Avoid eating lots of sweets. Sweets can quickly use up all the nutrients your body needs for its functioning. If you run short of energy, you are more likely to need protein than sugar.

Becoming vegetarian without information is risky. One teenager I know went vegetarian by cutting out meat and eating mostly white pasta. Instead of consuming good sources of plant protein, she propped up her flagging energy level with lots of coffee—not a diet to thrive on! Aware vegetarianism, on the other hand, can be a tremendously healthy way to eat.

Vegetarian travellers can source restaurants around the world on the net at: www.vegdining.com. The Toronto Vegetarian Association, North America's largest, offering a bimonthly newsletter, annual food fair, and resource center is at www.veg.ca.

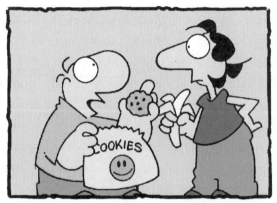

"Being a vegetarian isn't so bad.
For breakfast I had coffee and donuts,
for lunch I had corn chips and cola."

78. EAT MORE VEGETABLES.

Did you know there are people who think a vegetable is the pickle on their burger? If this astonishing statement is even partly true, it goes a long way towards explaining why laxatives are so popular. Without the fiber in vegetables to help move it through your system, meat sits in your intestines and rots. White flour products like bread or hamburger buns turn to glue.

Every single health expert I have read recommends eating plenty of vegetables. Some even go as far as to say the biggest food group in the ideal diet should be fresh, preferably organic, vegetables.

Not only do vegetables provide vitamins, minerals, enzymes, fiber, and water, they help the body to eliminate chemical toxins. Their antioxidants protect you from the free radicals which damage cells and genetic material and inhibit the immune system. They also help clear out the heavy metals you ingest from pollution. Many healing regimes rely on freshly-made vegetable juices as the main ingredient for cleansing and restoring the body.

Vegetables act as anti-cancer, anti-pollution, pro-digestion devices inside you, as long as you eat them fairly close to their natural state. Deep-frying, cooking in batter or smothering with butter or heavy sauces are not healthy ways to eat your vegetables.

But you don't have to steam all your vegetables, either. Annemarie Colbin points out that the slightly bitter, dark leafy greens like chard, kale, collards, and mustard greens taste better and are probably more nutritious when boiled for 10 minutes and drained. The longer cooking time softens and sweetens these vegetables, eliminating some of the oxalic acid they contain which makes more of their calcium available.

If you don't like the taste of many vegetables, try buying the organically-grown version. Commercially-grown vegetables sometimes taste bitter because of chemical residues or bland because they are grown in denatured soil—which also means their vitamin and mineral content is reduced. You may be surprised to discover you like the taste of the real thing when it's full of the flavor and richness of the true vegetable.

In *The Power of Superfoods*, Sam Graci recommends eating as many different colors of vegetables as you can every day. By doing so, you will ingest a full range of vitamins and minerals. My only caution here is that some vegetables contain calcium antagonists: spinach, kale, beet greens, and chard. Others are high in alkaloids which may interfere with calcium levels in the body: tomatoes, potatoes, green peppers, red peppers, and eggplant, also known as the nightshade group. You're better to eat these together at the same meal, leaving the calcium-rich vegetables to other meals, so you can absorb as much vegetable-source calcium as possible.

In the new food guides, grains tend to be the largest recommended food group, yet grains do not contain the nutrient, water, and fiber values present in vegetables. Grains are largely fuel. If you're very active, you'll burn them off. If not, you'll do better eating vegetables and fruit as the carbohydrates in your food plan. Carbohydrates are not just starchy foods. They are plant-source foods that are not primarily protein or fat. Vegetables, fruits, and grains all fall into this category.

To get more veggies into your meals, try a day of substituting vegetables for grains. For example, if you typically have a sandwich at lunch, put your sandwich filling on slices of cucumber, carrot and celery sticks, a mound of sprouts or chopped lettuce, or wrap it up in lettuce leaves. Make a bag full of raw veggies: cucumber, carrot, celery, radishes, parsley sprigs, fresh peas, sprouts, and baby salad greens and snack on them instead of chips, candy, cookies or popcorn. Bake sweet potatoes or squash to go with your dinner instead of potatoes or rice. Instead of pasta, put your sauce on finely chopped collard greens, or a bed of spaghetti squash, or a mixture of steamed or stir-fried veggies.

And if you don't have time or can't stand cooking vegetables, just grab whatever is easiest from the vegetable stand. Bags of prewashed baby carrots or boxes of alfalfa, red clover or green pea sprouts make great snacks or fast veggies to add to a meal. Celery and English cucumber are simple and quick: just rinse and chop. For a salad, grab a bag of prewashed baby salad greens. A box of any kind of sprouts makes a super-fast salad—just dump them on a plate and add some dressing.

It takes time to change dietary habits, so follow a pace that feels comfortable to you. Even if you eat *one* more vegetable than usual in addition to your regular food every day, you'll be doing yourself a big favor.

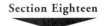

CALCIUM

79. WHY IS CALCIUM SUCH A BIG DEAL AND HOW MUCH IS ENOUGH?

Calcium is vital. There is more of it in your body than any other mineral, mostly in your skeleton, and it is used in all kinds of physical functions. Calcium helps form and maintain bones, teeth, and gums. It helps regulate heartbeat, transmit nerve impulses, maintain cardiovascular health and blood clotting, and activate enzymes which regulate metabolism and break down fats. It assists with growth and contraction of muscles and cell-wall permeability so nutrients move into and out of cells. Calcium inhibits the absorption of lead! It helps you assimilate iron, maintain your blood's acid-alkaline balance, and sleep well. Calcium is a factor in the prevention of osteoporosis and receding gums. According to Balch and Balch, it is also a factor in the protein structuring of DNA and RNA.

These days, nobody needs convincing about the importance of calcium. But how much is enough?

In some countries, people regularly consume only about 200 to 500 milligrams of calcium per day. North Americans, particularly pregnant and post-menopausal women, are encouraged to eat well over 1,000 milligrams by focussing on dairy products and supplements.

And does it work? Does all this emphasis on calcium make for better health? It doesn't look that way. North Americans have more heart, circulatory, dental, and bone loss (osteoporosis) problems than people who live in countries where the diet is more "primitive" and *lower* in calcium! If calcium alone were the deciding factor, the reverse would be true.

Clearly, there's more to the calcium question than simply how much you ingest. In North America, the focus tends to be on how you can *eat* as much calcium as possible. This may not be the optimal focus. What you really need to look at is, first, how can you best *absorb* the calcium you need? And, second, how can you prevent your body from *losing* calcium?

80. CALCIUM: ABSORB IT, KEEP IT.

To absorb calcium well, you need to:
1) reduce your stress
2) eat a balanced diet and avoid poorly tolerated foods
3) be careful with foods that contain calcium antagonists or inhibitors
4) get some natural sunlight every day

1) Stress is probably the number one inhibitor of all bodily functions, including absorption of minerals. No matter how good the food you eat, if you're over-stressed, you won't absorb nutrients well. Pausing to relax before eating, or practicing meditation or another relaxation technique will help.

2) Calcium is so important nature put it into a huge variety of foods. When you select your diet from as many food families as possible, you can't help but ingest this mineral.

But when you're intolerant or sensitive to certain foods, your body will absorb fewer nutrients from them no matter how many vitamins or minerals they contain. This is a good reason to find out if you react to any foods.

3) There are two groups of foods that contain calcium inhibitors and antagonists. The first group contains large amounts of phosphorus, concentrated sugars or alkaloids. They can help you develop arthritis, asthma,

cavities, obesity, glandular exhaustion and misfunction, dehydration, digestive problems, fatigue, malnourishment (because they use up the body's nutrients to be processed and eliminated), headache, behavior and learning problems, osteoporosis, and compulsive or addictive eating patterns. Yipes! This group includes carbonated beverages, caffeine, chocolate, nightshade vegetables (tomatoes, potatoes, green peppers, red peppers, and eggplant), sugar and sugar-sweetened foods, and tobacco. They are best avoided completely or consumed only on occasion.

The second group of foods contains the calcium antagonist oxalic acid. These foods can and should be eaten because of their other nutritional values *but not at every meal.* They are soy products, kale, spinach, rhubarb, beet greens, chard, almonds, and cashews. Eat these foods in moderation, once a day or less. Or restrict several to the same meal rather than spreading them out over the day. For example, mix almonds or cashews into a spinach salad, rather than eating the nuts and the vegetable at separate meals. Or have soy milk (or soy whip) with rhubarb pie rather than having the soy milk at breakfast and the pie at dinner. Be sure the other meals eaten that day contain good sources of calcium.

Annemarie Colbin explains you can free up much of the available calcium in dark leafy greens—kale, spinach, chard, and beet greens—by boiling them for several minutes to cook out the oxalic acid. Discard the cooking water. Blanched almonds (almonds with the skin removed) likewise will have more available calcium as the oxalic acid is in the skins, not in the nutmeat.

4) Natural sunlight is vital to calcium absorption. In countries where women wear full body veils that cover even their faces and eyes, osteomalacia or rickets (softening of the bones) is common. Your body uses the sunlight on your skin to make vitamin D, and vitamin D helps you assimilate calcium. Supplemental vitamin D does not function quite the same as what you produce yourself and is less effective, but it's better than nothing if you're not getting enough light during the day.

The best way to ensure enough vitamin D is to spend some time outdoors every day, *without* sunscreen or sunglasses. Some sunscreens interfere with the production of vitamin D. Judge the amount of time you plan to spend by time of year, time of day, and geographic location. You can still receive natural light on your skin while wearing a hat, sitting in the shade or on a cloudy day. Just make sure your eyes and some of your skin—face, arms or legs—are uncovered. Our ancestors ran around outdoors for thousands of years without sunglasses or sunscreen, and they had better bones than we do (according to British archeologists who dug some of them up.)

If you always wear sunglasses, slowly get used to going without them. Use protective lenses for extreme conditions like those that occur when skiing, boating or flying an airplane on a brilliant day. Overwearing of sunglasses can *make* your eyes light-sensitive. It takes time to restore your natural ability to cope with light, but it's always possible. Shade your eyes with a hat or visor instead.

Does sun really help with the absorption of calcium? Dr. Jacob Liberman and other researchers into the health benefits of natural light think so. They point out that your eyes need a daily dose of sunlight to stimulate your immune system, as well as for nutrient absorption.

What about keeping calcium in your body instead of losing it? You lose calcium like this: any food or drink that acidifies your bloodstream requires minerals, particularly calcium, to restore your body to its acid-alkaline balance. The calcium is dissolved from your bones and teeth, and is then lost from your body. (Sounds like osteoporosis, doesn't it?)

Foods that produce this effect are high in protein, fat, sugars, and salt. Nancy Appleton, Ph.D., author of *Healthy Bones*, says it can take more than 24 hours to return to homeostasis after eating sugar. Soft drinks and coffee inhibit your absorption of calcium and wash minerals right out of your body. Then there's wine and alcohol, vinegar, caffeine, and citrus fruits. Most of these foods are best avoided, especially by children. Foods and drinks that use up your minerals and make your blood acidic contribute to many health problems, especially bone loss and joint pain, so you may want to keep them to a minimum.

To counteract some of the negative effects, eat lots of alkalinizing foods. For example, a large serving of vegetables will balance the demineralizing effect of high protein foods. Leafy greens are especially good. Other alkalinizing foods are fruits, sea vegetables (seaweed), and sea salt. Annemarie Colbin points out that deep breathing also helps to alkalinize the system. Pure water is a balancing drink.

Finally, if you're concerned about osteoporosis, don't smoke. Smoking eats up your calcium, causing mineral malnutrition (to say the least). A study of people with osteoporosis that showed 75% of them were smokers.

81. WHAT ABOUT DAIRY?

Cows put on hundreds of pounds to mature. Unlike humans, calves attain a weight of about 300 pounds in their first year. To help them grow this big this fast, their mothers' milk contains huge amounts of protein and calcium.

When you ingest cow's milk or dairy products, you take into your body a substance meant to provide a huge growth spurt—to a *calf*. The nutrients in cow's milk are not in the correct ratio for humans. Our infants actually need more carbohydrate and fat in mother's milk than cattle require.

Although there is endless controversy over this, there is evidence that many adults and children have trouble digesting dairy. Milk is essentially baby food and we are the only species who continue to drink it after weaning. We are also the only species who regularly consume the baby food of *another* species. Every mammal's milk is composed so that it fosters the growth and development needs of *that species*.

After infanthood, most of us apparently do not retain the enzymes necessary to digest mother's or any other milk. There is a handful of populations who are genetically prone to retaining these enzymes, but they seem to be the exceptions on the globe. They are (far) Northern Europeans, vegetarian Hindus, and Berber tribes. For the rest of us, it's considered *normal* and it's certainly very common to have problems with milk and dairy products. John Lee, M.D., observes that pasteurization kills the natural enzymes in milk that make it digestible. Perhaps the populations who can digest dairy products in adulthood do not pasteurize their milk.

Dairy foods are any product that comes from the milk of a cow, goat or sheep. They include all cheeses, yogurt, ice cream, butter, cottage cheese, sour cream, cream, some forms of acidophilus, powdered milk, whey solids or powder, lactose, lactose-reduced or lactose-removed milk products, evaporated milk, and so forth.

Eggs are not a dairy food, even though they appear in the same department in the grocery store. They are the ovum of a chicken.

Annmarie Colbin, Anthony Sebastian, M.D., and Doris Rapp, M.D., among other researchers and doctors, relate dairy to an astonishing multitude of problems. Childhood ear infections are reported to be a common outcome of dairy consumption, as are allergies, skin and digestive problems, diarrhea, gas, and any mucus-related symptom such as stuffy or drippy nose, post-nasal drip, and chronic coughing and throat-clearing.

Because dairy is considered mucus-forming, many professional singers avoid dairy products—they cannot afford to cough or clear their throats in the middle of a solo. Dairy has been implicated in asthma, migraines, P.M.S., menstrual problems and infertility, and linked to juvenile-onset diabetes, as well as bed-wetting, diaper rash, colic, hardening arteries (even in children), and kidney stones. Hyperactivity and other behavior problems may be milk-related. The most ironic of health problems related to dairy is osteoporosis!

Can this be?! Milk, after all, is a wonder food. How can it be a factor in all these problems? Studies continue to reveal dairy as the top food allergen. Some authorities put it second to corn, however, since cows *eat* corn, you may end up with the problems of both allergens when you eat dairy products.

Cow's milk is higher in protein, calcium, and sodium than necessary for human needs. When you ingest all this excess, your body has to eliminate what you don't use. If your organs of elimination are at all stressed, or you force them to deal with the same excesses day after day, they will clog up and show symptoms of distress.

Pasteurization, homogenization and fortification of milk with vitamin D can also make trouble for human health. These processes change the milk molecules, affecting assimilation and digestion and the depositing of calcium into tissue instead of bone. If you have access to fresh, clean, raw (unpasteurized, unhomogenized, non-fortified) cow or goat milk and cheese, you may find you tolerate this better than any other type of dairy. Raw goat's milk is a good choice for infants who cannot be breast-fed.

What about dairy as a source of calcium? Well, it *is* a good source. For a cow. For humans, however, research shows dairy may not be so good. Dairy contains high levels of sulfur amino acids, which cause the body to excrete calcium! Cow's milk has an almost one-to-one ratio of calcium to phosphorus, and humans need a ratio more like two-to-one. These higher levels of phosphorus bind with calcium in the intestines and prevent it from being absorbed and assimilated into the body.

This is why dairy products may be a factor in osteoporosis. You *think* you're getting lots of calcium, because the nutrient charts show that dairy products contain high levels of the mineral. The only problem is, your body can't always access it. Anyone who reacts with intolerance to milk products absorbs few nutrients from them.

Milk and dairy products are often contaminated with high levels of antibiotics, commercial growth hormone, pesticides, and fertilizers from residues in the animals' feed or on pasturage. Toxins concentrate in fat cells and milk is full of fat. There is some concern that high fat and toxin levels in dairy are a factor in breast cancer.

If you're going to stick with dairy products, look into organically-produced versions. Susun Weed, author of *Menopausal Years The Wise Woman Way* thinks high-quality yogurt is an excellent source of easily digested calcium, to be eaten in moderation. Annemarie Colbin recommends avoiding dairy except on special occasions—holidays and parties. Moderation is always wise with controversial substances, as is seeking out the products that are least contaminated, processed, and bio-engineered.

82. CALCIUM SOURCES.

So, now that you know what *not* to eat, what are *good* sources of calcium? Pretty well all leafy green vegetables are good sources, particularly if they are organically grown. Calcium-rich vegetables include asparagus, broccoli, cabbage, collard greens, dandelion greens, mustard greens, parsley, turnip greens, watercress, and all lettuces. Other foods with high levels of calcium are figs, prunes, oats, hazelnuts, sesame seeds, sesame butter or tahini, carob, and most sea vegetables—dulse, kelp, wakame, nori, hijiki. Canned sardines or salmon with bones are also calcium sources.

You can make a calcium-rich herb tea by mixing together equal parts of nettle, red clover, raspberry leaf, oatstraw, and horsetail or any combination of these herbs (nettle is especially good). Use an ounce of herbs (about 15 tablespoons) to a quart or liter of water and let it steep for four hours to really draw the nutrients out of the herbs. Herbalist Susun Weed observes that a cup of this type of four-hour infusion gives you as much calcium as a cup of milk. It tastes good hot or cold.

To have sufficient calcium in your life, eat and drink calcium-rich items every day while avoiding the factors that make you lose calcium or keep you from absorbing it well.

Supplements:

Concerned that food cannot provide enough of what you need? Calcium supplements are controversial, as there is evidence to show they are not well absorbed. The calcium they provide may be deposited in the wrong places—in soft tissue rather than bone. Nancy Appleton cites research showing that women who take calcium supplements have no increase in bone density. These supplements may reduce iron in the body. If you go for food sensitivity testing, take along your calcium supplements and find out if they agree with you.

If you decide to take supplements, take small amounts of calcium over the day, with meals and at bedtime. This nighttime dose is thought to be absorbed best and may help prevent insomnia. Antacids are *not* a good calcium supplement. They bind phosphorus, create a mineral imbalance, often contain toxic levels of aluminum, and lack magnesium—a necessary cofactor in calcium absorption. Cofactors help you absorb the calcium well. Look for a supplement that contains cofactors such as magnesium, boron, manganese, vitamin C, and vitamin D (or sunshine).

The best way to supplement your calcium is with a whole food nutrient complex, as opposed to the isolated mineral on its own. Supplementary alfalfa, available in tablet form or liquid (or you can eat the sprouts), is a good source of calcium and other minerals. Kelp tablets are another such source, but should be used with caution by people with thyroid problems because of their high level of iodine. Green drinks like Pure Synergy, a mixture of organically-grown and wildcrafted ingredients, or Udo's Choice Beyond Greens will nourish your whole body, providing much more than additional calcium.

Don't forget some weight-bearing exercise to build your bones, and your daily dose of sunshine, so you can make lots of natural vitamin D and absorb your calcium.

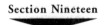

BREAD, PASTA & CEREAL GRAINS

83. FLOUR PRODUCTS & CEREAL GRAINS. ARE YOU OVER-EATING THEM?

Do you eat cereal and foods made with flour every day? Do you eat them at every meal and snack? It's not hard to do. After all, wheat is the predominant grain in the Western diet, followed closely by corn.

Wheat and corn are grass grains, along with oats, rice, rye, kamut, spelt, teff, wild rice, and millet. Grass grains are part of a botanical family that provides the basic carbohydrate ingredient for the huge number of food products made with flour, semolina, bran, durham, corn meal and/or corn sweeteners. Eat grass grains at every meal and you can quickly have too much of this food family.

Overeating of the grass grain family is one reason cereal and flour-food sensitivities develop. Another is that many people react to the gluten in grains. Elaine Gottschall, author of *Breaking the Vicious Cycle*, shows how bowel conditions including colitis, celiac disease, diarrhea, and Crohn's disease clear up when gluten-containing grains are removed from the diet for a period of time.

Even people with no allergies can react to grass grains without knowing these foods are the source of their problems. Chronic reactions include coughing, runny nose, indigestion, intestinal gas, diarrhea, constipation, skin problems, unexplained fatigue, menstrual problems, headaches including migraine, and hay fever. Mold is in some grains, according to A. Constantini, M.D., who studied fungal foods and their effects for the World Health Organization. Doris Rapp, M.D., cites mold and fungus as underlying stresses in asthma and many other health problems, particularly those with neurotoxic effects that trigger learning and behavior problems, depression, fatigue, anxiety, and emotional reactions.

Grain sensitivity can begin in infancy. Apparently, humans do not develop the enzymes to digest grains until after the age of six months. A child fed rice pabulum, formula, cereal or baby cookies containing grain or some type of grass grain sweetener (dextrose, corn syrup) too young is likely to develop a permanent intolerant reaction.

An easy way to discover if you are over-eating grains is to write down everything you eat for three days in a row. At the end of this time, compare your food record to the lists of grass grain-containing foods in the last two paragraphs of this chapter. This will quickly show you how often you eat grass grains and whether you are focussing primarily on a few food products and only one or two types of grain.

Food products made from conventionally rather than organically grown grains tend to be low in nutrients. Low nutrient foods are easy to overeat because your body will keep asking for the nutrients that are missing, making you think you're still hungry.

Grass grain flours are the basis for bread, rolls, pastries, cake, pie, cookies, doughnuts, muffins, pancakes, pizza dough, all the packaged mixes for making these items at home, cereal, crackers, bagels, all types of pasta, pretzels, pita, tortillas, croutons, bread crumbs, cones for ice cream, tacos, corn chips, and corn bread. Other food products containing grass grains are gravies and soups (especially cream soups), wafer or cookie-type chocolate bars, some potato chips and packaged peanuts, hotdogs, luncheon meats, salami, bologna, soy sauce, teriyaki sauce, foods cooked in batter—fish and fish sticks, chicken, tempura, etc., and most deep-fried foods other than french fries. (Of course, not *all* potato chips, peanuts, and hotdogs contain grains but you have to read the label to find out.)

Grain-derived sweeteners or thickeners may be listed on labels as dextrose, maltodextrin, corn extract, corn malt, corn syrup, flour, corn starch, and modified food starches. They are used in pasta sauce, peanut butter, salad dressing, cooked ham, and some canned baked beans, hotdogs, sausages, luncheon meats, instant soup powders and cubes, fruit drinks, mint jelly, pasta mixes, canned spaghettis, barbecue and other meat sauces, puddings, and fruit tart glazes. Corn is in some glues, so if you react to it, be careful about licking stamps and envelopes!

84. TRY A GRAIN-FREE WEEK.

Long ago, when the Pharoahs ruled, Egyptian wheat was one of the most nutritious foods available. Grown organically in the flood plains of the Nile, it was super-rich in minerals and vitamins. In some ways, it contributed to the growth of Western civilization. Today, wheat, like many foods, is often grown in nutrient-poor soils, may have been fed to you before you developed the enzymes to digest it, and could be creating unrecognized reactions in your body.

Wheat reactions mean different things to different people. I didn't think wheat affected me until I stopped eating it; then I found out I did react to it. A *lot*. I felt tired and mentally unfocussed and had digestive trouble when I ate wheat. Cell science researcher Elaine Gottschall links wheat and other grains to neurological disorders and such severe digestive and bowel problems as colitis, diverticulitis, and chronic diarrhea.

While eating wheat, I noticed other problems including a constantly running nose and menstrual cramps. A friend of mine finds her eczema and burning skin problems go away when she stops eating wheat. Another develops headaches or migraines several hours or a full day after she eats wheat. This is purely anecdotal evidence, but you can try a little experiment and find out how wheat and grains affect *you*.

If you're going to try this, you have to leave grains *completely* out of your diet for a full week. Be careful to avoid grains in *any* form. See the list of foods in the previous chapter if you're not sure what they're in, and *read labels* before you eat something. Your experiment will go better if you stay away from beer, rye whisky, and other beverages made from a grain base. Avoiding grains can be a challenge, so make things easy on yourself by assembling favorite foods that do not contain grains and have them available to munch on during your grain-free week. Choose from fruit and dried fruit, nuts, potato chips, cheeses and yogurt for those who tolerate dairy, any protein foods such as fish, meat or chicken (not luncheon meats), and all vegetables.

You may experience temporary symptoms and cravings while your body clears out the grain residues. These symptoms might include headaches and tiredness, so drink purified water and rest, whenever possible. Be careful around the fourth or fifth day, when the worst cravings tend to surface—usually just before they go away completely. If you're dying for a piece of bread, that's a clue to a possible wheat problem. You'll often crave the foods you react to most. Addictive eating of one grain can be a sign of food intolerance and related problems.

At the end of your grain-free week, eat only one bite of bread or other wheat-containing food. Now you will experience your body's *true reaction*. There are many possible reactions, including alterations in behavior and emotions—moodiness, depression, lack of focus, irritability, and inability to get going on tasks or projects, as well as physical reactions of indigestion, gas, runny nose, sneezing, headache, coughing, itchy skin, and unexplained tiredness. Do not eat more than one bite of the wheat food until you know how you react to it.

Be alert to *delayed* reactions. Doris Rapp, M.D., observes that skin problems such as eczema may take hours or a couple of days to develop. If you eat the wheat product in the morning, you might find you have a headache in the evening or the next day, or a sudden feeling of exhaustion, despite a full night's sleep. For this reason, it's best to reintroduce the wheat on a weekend.

However, *if you have eaten any food containing wheat during the grain-free week, you will not experience your body's true reaction.*

You can try the same thing with corn on another week. Or you can be tested for sensitivity by a professional. See chapter on *Testing for Sensitivities*.

Is it worth knowing your body's true reaction to wheat or corn if it's going to be painful? Absolutely! This knowledge gives you an incredible health advantage. Knowing how you react to grains will tell you if your body treats them as toxins. All toxins stress the immune system and contribute to your degeneration and disease potential.

For me, staying off wheat resolved some physical symptoms. It also made a surprising difference to my quality of life in terms of subtle responses such as clearer thinking, feeling more energetic, and easily staying awake and alert. An occasional piece of bread or dish of wheat pasta (there are other types) may be fine, it's the eating-wheat-every-day-at-every-meal syndrome that gets you into trouble.

People who are primarily sensitive to chemical pesticide and fertilizer residues in commercial grain products can feel much better by switching to organic products. The best solution for everyone is to expand what you eat to include less commonly known grains, and to eat creatively, without relying on wheat and corn as daily staples. The next chapter will help you with this.

85. ACHIEVING GRAIN VARIETY.

Wheat, corn, oats, and rice are so familiar, they often seem like the only grains in existence. In fact, they are four of several available grains. The others are barley, rye, kamut, spelt, teff, wild rice, millet, amaranth, quinoa (pronounced keen-wa), and buckwheat or kasha. (In case you are wondering about bulgar, it's wheat.)

Most of these grains belong to the same botanical family as grass and contain varying levels of gluten. The exceptions are amaranth, quinoa, and buckwheat (or kasha.) These three non-grass grains are seeds from other plant families, yet they can be cooked and eaten the same way as any whole grain. They are also available as flours and, because they lack gluten, are usually well-tolerated by anyone who reacts to grass grains. The lack of gluten means they cannot be substituted one-for-one in recipes that are based on regular (wheat) flour. See the *Cookbooks* section after the Resource Guide for cookbooks containing alternative flour recipes.

Amaranth, buckwheat, quinoa, and other grains are available in natural foods stores and sometimes in the regular grocery store. Eating the grain whole, as opposed to in flakes or flour, generally provides the highest level of nutrition.

No time to cook whole grains? Don't worry! All kinds of products made from organically-grown grains are now available. You can buy breads, muffins, and pastas made from spelt, kamut or rice, cookies made with oat or rice flour, packaged cold cereals from a variety of grains, "instant" quinoa that cooks in 90 seconds for a hot breakfast cereal (anyone who likes oatmeal will enjoy this), even an ice cream substitute called Rice Dream, which contains no dairy and is made from rice.

Whole grains and grain-based products must be chewed well, not only because they are fibrous but because your saliva contains an enzyme needed for their digestion. When you wolf your meals, the salivary enzymes never get the chance to break down the carbohydrates and you end up with digestive problems.

Reading labels:

Wherever you buy your food, it's very important to read labels. If you are wheat and corn sensitive, be sure the organic quinoa pasta you buy does not contain corn. Wheat or corn is often an ingredient in multi-grain breads and cereals and other products containing more than two grains. Look for single grain products: puffed kamut or millet cereal, rice bread, spelt muffins or noodles, or products that contain two well-tolerated grains: cookies made with rice and oats, pasta of kamut and quinoa, etc.

Sugar as a grass grain:

Sugar is from the botanical family of grass grains, so if you're sensitive to one or more grains, you may also react badly to cane sugar. In the natural foods store, this can be listed as organic, unrefined, natural cane juice or cane juice crystals, but don't be fooled. It's still cane sugar (though without the chemicals in conventional white sugar). If you're corn-sensitive, watch out for food products containing corn sweeteners such as corn malt. Better choices tend to be barley malt, rice syrup, maple syrup, and honey.

Making changes:

Changing your diet to include more grains can be a challenge. For one thing, the taste of wheat is so familiar, it may take time to adjust to the taste of other grains. They simply do not taste the same as wheat, nor do they all cook and bake the same. And they're not as available in restaurants and fast-food eateries.

Experiment with the new flavors and cooking properties. Spelt and kamut flours work well in breads, muffins, and cakes, and can be substituted one-for-one in recipes calling for wheat flour. Whole oats, amaranth, and millet make delicious hot cereals, sweetened with a little maple syrup or cooked with fruit. Rice, quinoa, and kasha are good in savoury herbed and spiced side dishes. Barley and millet tend to be bland and can be mixed into casseroles and soups.

Whole grains are easy to cook. Except for amaranth, buckwheat (or kasha), and teff, wash grains before cooking to remove grain dust. To wash whole grains, put the grain in a large bowl. Fill with water to an inch above the grain. Swirl with your hand. Then pour off the water through a strainer, and repeat the process until the washing water is clear, or mostly clear (about 3-5 times).

Cook the same way as rice: boil two to three cups of water with a pinch of salt for every cup of grain you plan to cook. Vary the amount of water, depending on the grain and how chewy or mushy you want it. Use your filtered water.

For convenience, cook whole grains in quantity and freeze jars of leftover grain for future meals. Whole grains can be eaten as hot breakfast cereal or a side dish at lunch or dinner, the way you'd eat rice.

A sense of humor helps in adopting these new grains. Think of it as a culinary adventure. After all, most of these grains are staples in one culture or another, and have been around for centuries. If you like the cuisine of India, the Orient, Russia or the Middle East, you'll find lots of recipes that call for other types of grain. In fact, you might even end up preferring grain variety! The pay-off is a healthier body and less stress on your immune system.

86. A DELICIOUS, CALCIUM-RICH, GRAIN-FREE TREAT.

Calcium-Rich Carob Fudge
The carob, tahini, and dried fruits (especially prunes and figs) in this recipe are all good sources of calcium. If you buy organic dried fruit, you will avoid the sulphites used to preserve the conventional version.

1 cup carob powder
1 to 3 cups dried fruit: use prunes, apricots, dates,
figs or raisins (or any combination of your choice)
3/4 to 1 cup honey
1 cup tahini (sesame butter)
1 cup walnuts or chopped hazelnuts or sesame and sunflower seeds

Rinse dried fruit with boiling water to wash off mold or yeast. Chop dried fruit and nuts. Often, children will not notice the taste of the dried fruits in the fudge because of the stronger taste of honey and carob. This is a good way to sneak fiber into what tastes like a candy and to use calcium-rich dried fruits children might not otherwise choose.

Gently heat honey over low heat in a pot large enough to hold all ingredients. As soon as bubbles start to appear in honey, turn it down or off so it doesn't boil, and quickly stir in the carob powder. Add the chopped dried fruits and nuts and stir so they are completely coated with carob/honey mixture.

Now stir in the tahini. This may take some arm power, but mix well. If you are having too much trouble getting the tahini to blend with the other ingredients, turn a very low heat on under the pot briefly and continue mixing.

When the mixture is cool enough to handle, either: 1) Take it out in spoonfuls and form into balls. Store in layers, in jars or tins, with waxed paper or baking paper between each layer. Keep in fridge or freezer. Or 2) Press into shallow pan lined with baking paper and cut immediately into squares. (You may need a wet knife to cut this fudge.)

Variations:

Hazelnuts contain calcium, so you can substitute hazelnut butter for tahini, if you prefer it.

You can make this fudge with organic cocoa powder (see Resource Guide for sources), however, this will eliminate the calcium benefits. Still, if you love chocolate, making this recipe with it will give you a healthier candy than eating conventional chocolate bars. When substituting cocoa powder for carob powder, try hazelnut, almond or cashew butter rather than tahini. Do not substitute sugar for honey in this recipe.

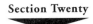

Sugar

87. SUGAR, VAMPIRE OF THE FOOD WORLD.

Sugar and sugary foods have been called "empty" calories. Actually, they're worse than empty, they're more like *vampire* calories. That's because sugar takes a lot out of the body and puts nothing back in but a quick buzz.

Wait a minute! Sugar must have *something* to offer. After all, what about that expression: "sugar is energy"? Well, it's true. Sugar is energy. But that's all it is.

This is how the equation works: calories = energy, sugar = calories, therefore sugar = energy. *And nothing else.* No vitamins, minerals, water, fiber, protein, EFA's or complex carbohydrates like in real food. The failure of sugar as a so-called food is that it offers no nutrients at all, not even enough to enable the body to metabolize it properly!

When you eat sugar, your body has to *cannibalize* its available vitamins and mineral stores, sacrificing bone, tooth, and joint integrity to keep itself in balance. These vitamins and minerals should be going into far more important physical processes like maintaining your set of teeth, healing cuts and bruises, maintaining proper neuron and brain function, and supporting the immune system to prevent degenerative conditions like arthritis.

Sugar sucks vitality from your body just to get itself digested, detoxified, and eliminated. That's why I think of sugar as vampire calories. The short-term energy sugar offers hardly seems worth having when its destructive effects are taken into account.

If you were to chew a piece of raw sugar cane at snack time, you'd get naturally-occuring, unconcentrated sugar juice, fiber, water, and some nutrients. Processing heats the cane and treats it with a list of frightening chemicals that not only destroy any vitamins and minerals but add toxins to the final product. The chemicals can include lime, carbon dioxide, calcium hydroxide, sodium carbonate, strontium hydroxide (which is radio active), sulphuric acid, and indathreme blue dye or ultramine (considered highly toxic). Physicians Randolph and Moss point out that sugar may contain microscopic particles of gas because of gas-fire reactivation of char filters. Anyone who is chemically sensitive can react negatively to these molecules.

In addition, processing takes the unconcentrated sugar juice in the cane and boils it down to a very concentrated sweetener that does not occur in nature. So much concentrated sweet is very hard for the human body to cope with, even after hundreds of years of exposure. Many health problems result. In *Sugar Blues*, William Dufty chronicles how, in the entire 400 years western civilization has been eating sugar as a regular part of the diet, no researcher has been able to find a single benefit to the human body! All results show the exact opposite—sugar leads to degeneration and disease. Even vampires won't eat it!

88. BUT I BRUSH MY TEETH SO WHY SHOULDN'T I EAT SUGAR?

Everyone knows about the connection between sugar and cavities. But the problems don't stop at your teeth. When you eat sugar, it inhibits your immune function for up to five hours afterwards, leaving you wide open to any passing virus or infection.

Sugars in any form accomplish this suppression of your immune response by slowing down the activity of the neutrophils, which make up much of your white blood cell count. The white blood cells are a large part of your immune system. So, if you happen to consume a sugar-sweetened cereal or pastry at breakfast, a soft drink at lunch, several cookies or lots of fruit juice for a snack, and dessert at dinner, your immune system is literally immobilized for the entire day!

This could play out for you in several ways. You might have trouble healing from bruises and cuts, catch colds easily, recover slowly from illness, repair broken bones with difficulty, or have frequent ear, nose, and throat infections. You may also find yourself suffering from chronic degenerative conditions. Sugar tends to exhaust the adrenal glands, putting you in a state of constant fatigue.

When sugars have such a powerful effect on the immune system, it's no wonder school children all come down with colds at the same time, particularly after high-sugar holidays like Christmas and Halloween.

Then there's the brain connection. Consider Dr. David Schweitzer's statement: "German researchers have learned that intelligence, measured in terms of the mental capacity to think, reason, and memorize, is *significantly reduced when sugar is consumed.*" (italics ours) In *Food and Healing*, Annemarie Colbin lists "hyperactivity, lack of concentration, depression, anxiety, psychological disorder, insanity, and even violent criminal behaviour" as possible results of a diet high in refined sugar.

But sugar affects far more than thinking capacity and behavior. Obesity, diabetes, and hypoglycemia are diseases associated with sugar consumption. Obesity has many dangerous outcomes from the stress it puts on the body. Diabetes can kill you. William Dufty links sugar to cancer and heart disease.

Hypoglycemia is a condition in which blood sugar levels fall below normal because of the oversecretion of insulin by the pancreas. Like candida, another sugar-related problem, hypoglycemia can mimic other diseases and is related to problems with allergies, digestion, and memory. It may *appear* to be a minor condition (compared to, say, the plague), but hypoglycemia is tremendously distressing for the sufferer, particularly as the symptoms are often misunderstood and put down to such causes as lack of self-control, laziness or psychological problems. And they can worsen with age!

Sugar is also considered to be a factor in myopia, high cholesterol, and in the "genetic narrowing of pelvic and jaw structures, crowding and malformation of teeth." When I spoke to a dentist about permanent teeth that do not grow in after baby teeth are removed, he casually told me it's quite common. Yet populations who live on "primitive" diets of whole foods that are not refined or processed tend to grow full sets of large, healthy teeth.

How much sugar is too much? Here's the kicker. Your body is not really equipped for eating any food that contains refined or processed sugars, except on rare occasions! In the past, this would mean feast days or holidays, which puts it at perhaps six to eight times a year, or, at *most*, once a month.

Everyone is better off with complex carbohydrates like whole grains, fruits, and vegetables. While the simple sugars in refined and processed foods shock your body with a sudden overdose of sugar, whole foods take time to digest, providing you with a slow, steady supply of glucose and allowing your brain and body to function in balance. When you get right down to it, sugar and sweets just don't make for good health, even if you brush your teeth.

89. IF YOU CRAVE SWEETS, DON'T BLAME YOURSELF. BLAME YOUR CHEMISTRY.

Note: The brain chemicals referred to in this chapter are not the same as synthetic (man-made) chemicals or petrochemicals. Brain chemicals or "neurotransmitters" are a natural part of your body. They help to transmit messages among cells.

Ever wonder why you keep right on craving sweets, even when you know they're not good for you? Is it your willpower that's at fault? Are you a hopeless sweetaholic?

Not according to Kathleen DesMaisons, Ph.D., author of *Potatoes not Prozac*, and Joel Robertson, M.D., who wrote *Natural Prozac*. They believe sweet craving has more to do with brain chemistry than will power.

Specifically, it's low levels of seretonin and beta-endorphin that make you crave sweets. Both of these feel-good brain chemicals help to reduce levels of pain, anxiety, depression, isolation, and negativity while raising self-esteem, tolerance, optimism, compassion, and ability to focus and concentrate.

Enough beta-endorphin can even make you euphoric!

You'd have to be crazy not to want more of these brain chemicals. But there are good and bad—healthful and harmful—ways to produce them in your body.

Dr. Robertson believes most of us are low in seretonin most of the time because of the high-stress lifestyle predominant in our culture. To counteract low seretonin, many of us typically eat sweets or drink coffee. These are the familiar, if unconcious, methods used to restore brain chemical and blood sugar levels.

Some people drink alcohol or use cocaine for the same reasons. Whether you turn to cocaine or coffee, the underlying motive is the same: stimulation of brain chemistry. And whether you choose drugs or alcohol, coffee or sweets, the result tends to be *over*stimulation. There are many downsides from overstimulation including addiction, adrenal gland exhaustion, weight problems, headache, depression, heart problems, emotional yo-yoing, and other physical and mental health concerns.

Instead of going to such extremes, you can stimulate your brain chemicals through various activities, according to both DesMaisons and Robertson. They list exercise, meditation and prayer, music, dancing, communing with nature, journaling about real emotions, and orgasm! Any activity that brings you joy makes all your cells healthier and will tend to reduce cravings for stimulants. Laughing works wonders.

To balance your brain chemicals as well as your cravings, eat regular meals of real (not junk) food. This is simple, old-fashioned advice, but it works! Include protein, vegetables, and fruit in your meals so your body has actual nutrients to work with, rather than relying on caffeine and pastries. Eat slow food, or the best quality fast food you can access. This may mean bringing your own sandwich and apple. You are less likely to crave sweets if you keep your blood sugar balanced with real food.

Other factors that may unbalance your neurotransmitters and homeostasis and lead to sweet craving are chemical exposure (another reason to buy toxin-free household and personal care products), an overgrowth of candida (may occur pre-period in some women), and excess metal in your mouth.

The suggestions in this book can help you reduce or eliminate these factors so you and your chemistry can work together to end sweet cravings.

90. SUGAR AND BLOOD SUGAR. WHAT'S THE DIFFERENCE?

If we haven't already said enough bad things about sugar, here's something else. Sugar does even more damage than its vampire trick of using up your vitamin and mineral supplies. It overstimulates the pancreas, which regulates blood sugar.

That may not sound very serious, but a disorder in blood sugar regulation can become diabetes, an often fatal disease. There are other less deadly but still troublesome effects of blood sugar imbalance.

Sugar—refined sugar and other sugars in our foods—is not the same thing as blood sugar. Blood sugar, or glucose, is the food of the brain and is manufactured *by the body* from the foods you eat. (There is also a glucose used as sweetener in food products but this type of glucose is made in a factory from starches like corn, rather than by your body.) Sugar is something you eat, and blood sugar is something your body produces. The body strives to keep a balanced level of blood sugar at all times.

When blood sugar is out of balance, everyone reacts differently, depending on genetics. You might feel hungry, tired, crabby or fuzzy-headed, unable to think properly or focus on what you're doing. Such regular activities as working on your computer, putting together a meal or trying to remember where you left your car keys become a major challenge when your blood sugar is off. Low blood sugar can bring on food cravings, anxiety, temper tantrums, even violent behavior!

Refined sugars convert very quickly to glucose. In fact, they convert so fast, they cause a rapid rise in blood sugar, making the level too high for your body's natural state of balance. In response, your pancreas floods the bloodstream with insulin to bring the blood sugar back down to its normal level.

Overeating of sugars can result in diabetes or hypoglycemia. Diabetics underproduce insulin and hypoglycemics overproduce it. Either way, both of these groups have trouble regulating their blood sugar and *eating* sugar is not the solution, since sugar is what creates the blood sugar imbalance in the first place.

If you are hypoglycemic, your body will respond to sugar jolts by producing *way* too much insulin, which brings the blood sugar level down too low! Then your body signals for a rise in blood sugar, to bring it back up to normal. This signal is often misinterpreted by you as a craving for another sweet. If you eat more sugar, you end up on the blood sugar/insulin roller coaster ride: blood sugar goes up too fast, too much insulin is produced, blood sugar goes down too fast, sweet craving, sweet eaten, blood sugar goes up too fast, and so on. It's a vicious cycle.

The only way out is to eliminate refined sugars, refined flour products, and caffeine from your diet, all of which overstimulate the pancreas. Instead, eat complex carbohydrates—vegetables, fruit, and whole grains. These foods release their sugars slowly while they are being digested, providing a slow, steady drip of glucose (blood sugar) instead of the high-voltage jolt of refined sugars. Eating a little protein with them can help, too.

Hypoglycemics often experience food cravings for high-sugar items, including alcohol, and many struggle with weight problems and eating disorders all their lives. Hypoglycemia in childhood can be a precursor to alcoholism in adulthood. It can also be the precursor to diabetes.

Diabetics cannot produce enough insulin to regulate excess sugar in the blood. Diabetes is a life-threatening condition, and, like hypoglycemia, is very much diet-related. In particular it is related to high sugar consumption. Among populations who do not eat refined sugar and processed foods, diabetes is unknown.

91. AIM FOR SWEET-FREEDOM.

If you change only one element of your diet, decide to eat less refined sugar or eliminate it completely from your life. Choosing sweeteners that are easier on the body will put you way ahead of the crowd in the level of health you enjoy, not only physically, but mentally and emotionally!

Prior to the 1500's, sweets were seldom available. Most people had the opportunity to eat sweets—usually sweetened with honey—and rich foods only on feast days. Then they went back to regular fare, which might include a little meat, fish or poultry, raw milk, cheese, whole grains and whole grain bread, and veggies and fruits in season.

We in the modern world can feast on rich and fatty foods *and* eat sugary sweets at any time, any day of the week. The result is our many "diseases of civilization". Sugar is so prevalent in our western diet, many of us eat it at every meal and snack, often without even realizing it is in the food we have chosen. The list of foods containing sugar is almost as long as the list of problems and diseases associated with it.

A glance at the labels on processed foods reveals sugar under several different names: sucrose, brown sugar, golden sugar, glucose, dextrose, dextrin, fructose, lactose, maltose, syrups, and any of these in combination. The constant availability of sweeteners makes it hard to believe there was actually a time when refined white sugar did not exist!

In fact, for most of human history, the only sweets available were honey and fruit and these were restricted by climate, season, luck, and wealth. People ate the plants and animals that lived in their own geographic location. Only when Europeans came to the New World and plantations began their slave-based production did sugar take its place in the western diet. (Not to mention chocolate and coffee.) Even after sugar became available, it took more than three hundred years to reach current levels of consumption at *over* 100 pounds per person per year!

Sugar consumption has skyrocketed in the 20th century, particularly in North America and England. According to D.S. Khalsa, M.D., author of *Brain Longevity*, about 25% of what most people eat is sugar and another 33% is fat, which means over 50% of the average diet is nothing but fat and sugar! No wonder North Americans struggle with obesity.

Processed "low-fat" foods made with sugar and other sweeteners do *not* make your diet less fattening. Udo Erasmus points out that *refined sugars and starches turn to fat in your body. Real* low-fat foods are fruit, vegetables, whole grains, fish, and poultry without skin. Artificial sweeteners are processed non-nutrients. There is concern that some may be carcinogenic and/or a factor in neurological disorders and other health problems.

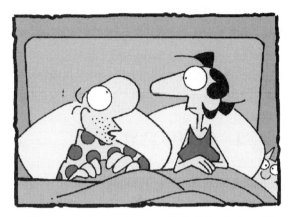

"I've got to quit my diet. My fat cells
kept me awake all night with
their protest march."

Sugar unbalances the body, prompting a compensatory demand for heavy doses of protein, but protein can only partially compensate for the damage sugar causes. According to Annemarie Colbin, strict vegetarians who consume honey and sugar set up dangerous protein deficiencies in their bodies, causing both physical and mental health problems. She cites the example of Hitler, a vegetarian who ate vast amounts of sugar and refined starch products but very little (plant) protein. His bizarre food habits could easily have contributed to his temper tantrums, behavior aberrations, and recurring violent nightmares. Certainly his diet was wildly unbalanced and did not contain the range of nutrients healthy vegetarians consume.

Nutrition studies with prison inmates show the behavior of violent individuals calms markedly when sugar and low-nutrient junk foods are taken out of their diets. The negative emotional and psychological consequences of eating sugar range from low self-esteem and forgetfulness to confusion, hallucinations, and even manic-depression!

Is it ever appropriate to eat sweets? After special meals. At a few parties and celebrations. Think of sweets as a stimulant like alcohol. If you're using every day, you're an addict.

Apart from the tremendous health benefits, perhaps the best reason to go sweet-free is this: when you don't eat sweets, you can taste and appreciate other foods properly. In the bad old days when I ate sugar, sweets were really all I wanted to eat. Now that I eat real food, I have much more appreciation for the whole world of flavors that exists outside of sugar. And every day I'm away from sugar makes it easier to live entirely without the stuff. Trust me!

92. TREAT YOURSELF TO THE BEST.

Does that mean rushing out and blowing your week's paycheque on a huge box of hand-made truffles? Not on your life! Lots of expensive chocolatiers still use refined white sugar full of chemicals and chocolate from plants heavily sprayed with pesticides.

Eating the best means eating the sweets that are the best quality for *your body*. The best quality sweets and sweeteners are lower in concentrated sugars and easier on the pancreas, brain, and immune system because they don't provoke a big blood sugar/insulin response, are not chemically produced, and contain healthier ingredients than most sugary sweets.

Ideally, fruit would be the sweetest item in your diet. But, if you're like me, it's not that easy to go straight from regular doses of white sugar and chocolate to nothing but fruit for dessert. After fruit, the next best sweets are baked goodies and frozen desserts made from whole grains, organically-grown ingredients, and high quality sweeteners. These sweeteners include unpasteurized honey, maple syrup, barley malt, rice syrup, stevia, fructose, and unrefined cane juice crystal products such as Sucanat and Rapidura. They can be found in natural foods stores either in bulk for cooking or as the sweetener in baked goods.

Concentrated fruit juice is used to sweeten some brands of cookies, fruit leathers, and fruit spreads (also known as jam, but for some industry reason, the word "jam" can't be used on the label of a spreadable fruit product unless it contains sugar!) Fruit juice-sweetened items are a great choice as they taste delicious but are less likely to trigger a problematic blood sugar response than are concentrated sweeteners.

Any concentrated sweetener eaten *in excess* will have the same effect on the body as sugar, overloading the pancreas (blood sugar/insulin response), adrenals, and immune system and creating a possible protein and mineral deficiency. Unrefined cane juice crystals, maple syrup, and honey are the most concentrated alternatives to sugar, so be careful with them. Cane juice crystals can have about the same effect as refined white sugar, despite the differences in processing. Honey is a monosaccharide or single sugar, unlike most other sweeteners, so it is easy to digest and is therefore preferred for anyone with digestive or bowel trouble.

Fructose is less concentrated than the three sweeteners mentioned above, and barley malt and rice syrup are the least concentrated, so will be less sweet and easier on your blood sugar. Stevia or honeyleaf is extremely sweet, requiring only about a quarter of a teaspoon to sweeten a recipe. Because it's an herb that tastes sweet rather than a concentrated sweetener, it may be better tolerated by sugar-sensitive people.

When you take refined sugar out of your diet, you will discover the natural sweetness of foods (in addition to fruit). Many vegetables, especially when organically grown, are surprisingly sweet: carrots, squash, parsnips, corn on the cob, beets, peas, and sweet potatoes in particular. Even organically-grown kale can taste sweet. Nuts are sweet too—try cashews, almonds, macadamias, pecans or uncolored pistachios (without the red dye). Oats, sweet rice, and amaranth are the sweeter grains.

If you're a sweet craver, check out what's available from the natural foods store and stock up so you won't be caught short in the middle of the night when the store is closed. Look for products that contain whole grains or fruit for fiber, high quality oil, and a little protein from soy or nuts. This will be a major change from the usual grocery product made from white flour, white sugar, and altered fats, all of which add up to glue in your intestines and a big toxic strain on your immune system. Try nut and seed bars sweetened with honey or Carob Rocky Choc, a delicious carob-coated crisped rice bar sweetened with honey and malt, from Sunfresh Organics.

If you love chocolate, buy chocolate bars or cocoa powder made from organically-grown chocolate. Use the cocoa powder for hot chocolate with soy or almond beverage and honey, or for baking brownies full of nuts and dried fruit which add protein and fiber to your sweet. There are many wonderful brands of organically-grown chocolate such as Fairtrade associates, Hawaiian Vintage Chocolate, Rapunzel, Terra Nostra, Pronatec, and Sunspire.

Try different brands of cookies sweetened with fruit juice, rice syrup or barley malt. Don't fall into the trap of buying everything sweetened with cane juice crystals. You can end up overdoing that one as easily as sugar. Look for frozen desserts—ice cream substitutes—made from fruit, soy, hemp or rice. Rice Dream, Soy Delicious, Cool Hemp (Cool Maple is maple-syrup sweetened), and Sweet Nothings are popular brands.

Think of your sweets in terms of how they might add to your health picture, instead of taking away from it. After I started to think this way and substituted high quality sweets for my old standbys, I noticed a major change. After I ate the healthier sweet, I felt...good! The sick feeling that can occur after sugary sweets was gone. Nor did I react with the usual swelling and tingling hands, unsettled stomach, indigestion, and zinging teeth.

Dentists and brain chemistry experts recommend eating sweets at the end of a meal when they will do the least damage to your teeth and your blood sugar levels. Eating sweets alone is worse than eating them with meals. If you crave a sweet for quick energy at other times of day, drink a glass of water first, in case you are tired due to dehydration. Eat a little protein before your sweet (a handful of nuts will do). This will help to stabilize your blood sugar and help to prevent a sweet-induced roller coaster ride.

COOKING & SHOPPING

93. COOKWARE THAT DOESN'T SCARE US.

In *Prescription for Nutritional Healing*, Balch and Balch point out that cooking in aluminum pots can increase the amount of aluminum in your food. Since a buildup of aluminum and mercury in the body is a recognized factor in Alzheimer's disease, I use stainless steel pots and pans. If you have the arm strength, you can try iron cookware. Glass—like Corningware or Pyrex—is another good choice. Stainless steel, iron, and glass will not leach tiny amounts of dangerous metals or other invisible ingredients into your food during the cooking.

Non-stick cookware is coated with a chemical. Does every single molecule of the chemical stay on the pot surface when it's heated? If it doesn't, it's getting into your food. If you happen to scratch the surface with a utensil while cooking, little particles of chemical are liable to break off and end up in your dinner.

To keep plastic molecules out of your food, don't cover it with plastic wrap before microwaving. Instead, put a paper towel over the food, or use a microwavable glass dish with its own (glass) lid. Microwave cooking is controversial because it alters food molecules, particularly protein. Very brief exposures may be okay. Reheating a drink in the microwave uses up more power than reheating it on the stove.

Go for glass measuring cups, wooden or stainless steel utensils, and glass baking pans. Muffin tins tend to be aluminum or non-stick coated, so if you know where to buy them in stainless steel or glass, write and let us know! In this case, you may have to rely on muffin papers to protect the muffins from the pan. Baking paper can be used on cookie sheets.

In general, my policy with cookware and utensils is that if I don't want it in my food, I don't cook with it.

94. PAY SOMEONE ELSE TO COOK YOUR STAPLES.

If you don't have a lot of time to cook, the easiest way to make sure you have lots of healthy food available in the house is to make big batches once a month or whenever you can and keep them in the freezer. Set aside a cooking day every so often to make large pots of whole grains, then put meal-sized portions into jars or cellulose bags and freeze them. Other foods that freeze well are casseroles, soups, whole-grain noodle lasagne, desserts, and fresh seasonal fruit and vegetables.

One friend buys large quantities of locally-grown organic vegetables in season, then blanches and freezes them in meal-size portions. All winter, she has a wonderful selection of delicious veggies that only need quick heating, saving her time and money.

A freezer full of organic, ready-to-warm food sounds great to you, but you don't have the time to make it? Hire someone, even your teenager, to spend several hours cooking up your freezer food and/or shopping for the ingredients. When the person is from outside your family, instead of having them cook for you at their house, it may be easiest to turn your kitchen over to them for several hours, so that all the ingredients, recipes, and jars for freezing will be available in one place. This provides some quality control for you. Show them how you like your foods prepared—using filtered rather than tap water, sea salt rather than iodized salt, stainless steel rather than aluminum pots, and have them label and date the jars so you know what's in them!

If you don't have time for any of the above but like to eat healthy food, and you live in an urban area, scan local health magazines and newspapers for cooking services. These usually deliver several day's selections of meals or dinners once a week to your home. You store them in your freezer and simply heat up the one you want. This way you always have meals available without having to prepare anything. No fuss, no muss. In our city, I've noticed many of these services are vegetarian—a good choice for people who want to eat lightly at dinner time.

95. EXPLORE A NATURAL FOODS STORE. READ LABELS.

If you have never shopped at a natural foods store, go to one or two to familiarize yourself with the layout and products without necessarily planning to buy anything. Some stores are better than others, containing a wider selection of goods or lower prices. Some sell nothing but vitamins, supplements, and power bars. Others sell bulk and packaged foods but do not carry fresh produce. Some are full service grocery stores specializing in organic foods.

If the first store you go to does not appeal to you, try another. Ask your friends who shop at natural foods stores which ones they recommend and why. Ask them to show you around their favorite store and point out products they like. Or talk to the staff in the establishment and have them show you what is available. Explain this is your first visit to such a store. Ask if most of the products are organic, if they sell non-irradiated herbs and spices, and how often produce comes in.

Stores with good organic produce sections usually receive fresh produce daily or almost daily. If you don't recognize all the vegetables, ask the produce manager what they are and how to cook them. Stores with poor organic produce have a slow turn-over of these goods. When there is only one natural foods store in your area, they may receive a produce delivery only once a week. Find out what day this is and shop for produce on that day or ask the proprietor to save fresh, good quality produce items for you until you can get to the store. (But play fair. Don't wait a week to pick up the produce and then refuse to buy it because it no longer looks fresh!) Many families buy an annual share in a Community Supported Agriculture (CSA) farm which provides them with organically or biodynamically grown produce all through the growing season.

A natural foods store may not be as big and bright as the typical chain grocery store in a shopping mall. Don't be put off. While natural foods stores are retail outlets and are in business to make money, they are usually started by people who have a commitment to health and/or environmental concerns and will reflect a philosophy that is based on more than simply moving large volumes of product off the shelves and into the consumer's grocery basket. The 'look' in a natural foods store can range from natural wood shelving and soft, ambient lighting to high-tech metal shelves and full-spectrum tube lighting. Perhaps the most consistent feature of natural foods stores is that each one will be unique. Because these stores tend to be more personal, my experience is that they restore the social aspect of shopping.

It's always a good idea to read labels on packaged foods, even in the natural foods store, so you know what's in the item you are buying. Not all foods are healthy or a good choice for *everyone* just because they are sold in a health food store. Here are some things you will learn when you read product labels. You will find out whether there are ingredients that disagree with you (check the list of allergens in chapter 4), whether there is a high proportion of sugars or cooked fats in the food (if it's a bakery product or it's on a shelf as opposed to in the refrigerated section, the oils are cooked) and whether or not the food actually contains any nutrients. How will you know if there are nutrients? Usually if a food product is made up of other *foods*, not just chemicals or words you can't pronounce, there's a good chance there will be some nutrition in it.

In the natural foods store, you'll find many alternatives to conventional milk, cheese, bread, ice cream, peanut butter, and other foods. Look for milk-substitute beverages made from soy, rice or almonds, soy or rice cheese-type products and goat cheeses, nut butters—almond, cashew, hazelnut, macadamia, pistachio, sunflower or tahini (sesame seed butter), and breads that are a change from wheat flour. Spelt raisin bread is a good one to start with, or choose plain spelt or kamut.

Instead of ice cream, pick up frozen desserts made from rice, soy or fruit such as Rice Dream, Soy Delicious or Sweet Nothings. To make life easier on your blood sugar, choose the versions that do not contain sugar or unrefined cane juice crystals. If your retailer does not carry them, ask that they order these products. Most natural foods stores welcome customer input and base some of their buying decisions on customer requests. At home, store nut butters, whole grain breads or muffins, and high-quality oils in the refrigerator or freezer as they contain no preservatives and will not last on the shelf the way chemically-treated products do.

If you need fast meals, look at the many types of quick or prepared foods, such as herbed and flavored rice, bean dishes, frozen pasta and dinners, soy patties and 'hot dogs', turkey franks, vegetable paté, and Middle Eastern hummus and salads. Ask the staff for help in finding any items. Once you have become familiar with these items, you may notice that some of them are available in the regular grocery store.

Introduce these new products slowly into your meals, as you use up foods currently in your kitchen and get used to new tastes. Many natural foods stores have deli counters where you can buy cooked dishes, salads, and other ready-made foods that will introduce you to unfamiliar grains and flavors you want to discover.

ENTERTAINMENT

96. PARTIES AND DINING OUT.

Is there such a thing as a healthy way to party or is the very idea a contradiction in terms?

In general, party refreshments lean heavily on many of the common food allergens: sugar, corn, wheat, dairy, caffeine, and alcohol. You can usually take in a good dose of altered fats at a party, in corn or potato chips, and some baked goods. And then there's smoke. (see the next chapter on *Smoking* for tips on ways to keep it from overloading your system.) On the other hand, nobody's perfect. Good health does *not* mean putting an end to your social life!

When you have generally good health habits, you can afford to indulge on occasion (unless you are ill.) Here are some tips on keeping indulgence from overloading you.

Before you go to a party or restaurant, choose your strategy according to your preferences and state of health. Are you a sweet lover? Do you love rich sauces? Or would you prefer a glass or two of good wine or a really decadent coffee? Choose your favorite "poison" and go with that, rather than blowing out on everything on the menu.

Have your wine or dessert with a plain meal: fish or chicken, veggies, and salad. Ask for olive oil to put on your salad instead of dressing which often contains sweeteners and poor quality toxic oils. Go for the baked potato rather than french fries which are deep-fried. If you like an elaborate entree, skip the wine and/or dessert. When coffee is your choice, remember that decaf may be processed with chemicals. Unless the decaf is organically-grown or Swiss water-processed (decaffeinated without chemicals), you may be better off drinking caffeinated coffee on occasion.

When you're going to a wedding and you know there will be a big gap between the service and the reception, bring your own healthy snack —a bag of nuts and a piece of fruit will do it—or eat something beforehand. This will stabilize your blood sugar until the meal is served and keep you from falling on the hors d'oeuvres like a starving wolf. Hors d'oeuvres vary wildly in ingredients but many contain one or more of the most common reactive foods (wheat, dairy, sugar, processed meats), and may be deep-fried or otherwise contain altered fats. The meal itself is usually a better choice. When the hors d'oeuvres consist of simple foods such as fresh vegetables, fruit, and plain protein (salmon, chicken, shrimps, hummus, marinated tofu), pig out.

At parties, choose vegetables over chips or crackers to put dips and cheeses on, especially if you have bowel or digestive trouble. If you suspect there will be nothing you can eat at a party, bring a vegetable tray, or a bag of organic corn chips and some organic hummus or salsa. When you're not feeling completely well, or everyone in your office or school has a cold, decide to avoid sweet foods and drinks. Viruses take a few days to incubate and sweets can inhibit your immune system for up to five hours after eating or drinking them, which is enough time for a virus to get a good grip on you. Instead of immobilizing your immune system with birthday cake, take a piece home with you and freeze it until you're feeling better and the flu bug has gone to another office building.

When you plan to drink alcohol or eat sugar-sweetened anything on an evening out, eat some protein first. Supplements I have found useful are chromium picolinate to help stabilize my blood sugar, milk thistle to help clear my liver, zinc, B-complex vitamins, vitamins C and E, and enzymes.

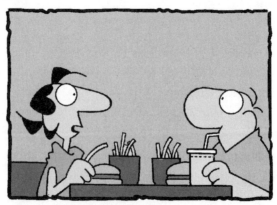

"No, the lumps in your milkshake do not count as fiber."

These nutrients and antioxidants may help to counteract the effects of alcohol and sugar as well as the dangerous free-radical effects of junk food and foods made with altered and cooked fats.

Nutritional supplements and fresh vegetables are two sources of helpful antioxidants. Red wine is a third. Red wine is perhaps less harmful than other types of alcohol, unless you react to sulphites or are allergic to alcohol. If you are grain-sensitive, you may find wine is easier on you than grain-based beer or liquors such as rye or scotch. Organic wines are available in most liquor stores; ask store staff about them. Bring a bottle of your own high-quality water to a party so you can alternate alcoholic beverages and water.

Some people like to "sober-up" with coffee at the end of an evening, however, both alcohol and caffeine are dehydrating. If you have drunk these (hopefully not too often!), drink water when you get home and on the following day to rehydrate your body. You may also wish to take another dose of supplementary vitamins and minerals, or plan to drink freshly made fruit and vegetable juices the next day to restore nutrients and hydration. A morning-after drink made with Pure Synergy or Beyond Greens nutrient powder could help.

Finally, if you live perfume- and smoke-free, but the outing is in a perfumy, smoky environment, wash your hair when you get home, or if it's too late for that, wrap a towel around your head to cover your hair so you won't have to breathe the smoke and scent fumes that have stuck to it, while you sleep. Leave your party clothes to air in a room other than your bedroom or out on your balcony, so you can sleep chemical-free.

97. SMOKING.

There are about 4,000 chemicals and over 40 known carcinogens in cigarette smoke. But smokers don't need to worry too much about dying of cancer, since the majority of them die from heart problems.

If you *live* with a smoker, go ahead and worry. Those thousands of toxic chemicals can affect nearby non-smokers as much as, if not more than, the smokers themselves. Children, with their developing immune systems, are even more sensitive to the toxins in second-hand smoke than adults.

Problem substances in cigarettes can include cyanide, carbon monoxide, radioactive particles, nitrogen dioxide, vinyl chloride, cadmium, and ammonia. Tobacco smoke has been linked to lowered immunity, cancers, leukemia, reduced mental abilities, miscarriage and stillbirth, sudden infant death syndrome, asthma and bronchitis, heart and circulatory problems, impotence and sterility in males, osteoporosis and early menopause, incontinence, vitamin deficiency, rapid aging, and injury to DNA.

If *you* live with a smoker, here are a couple of things you can do to protect yourself and other non-smokers in the household, including pets. Ask smokers not to smoke indoors. If they turn you down, they may be persuaded to smoke beside an air filter machine which will help to clear *some* of the toxins from smoke-filled air. Smokers who only smoke outside the home can change into smoke-free clothes when they come home to non-smokers, since smoke sticks to clothes. Even the smell of it can affect those who are smoke-sensitive, particularly children.

Vitamin supplementation is another possibility for protection of smokers and their housemates. Vitamins C, B complex and E, and coenzyme Q10 (Co-Q10) are important as antioxidants to protect cells and cellular processes from smoke damage. Zinc is vital. Without it, the cadmium in cigarette smoke will lodge in the body's receptors where zinc belongs. Over time, excess cadmium damages kidneys and raises blood pressure.

Vitamin A helps to protect lungs and mucous membranes. Eating *lots* of organically grown fruits and vegetables, especially leafy and green vegetables, will help clear chemicals and heavy metals out of the body. Kelp, alfalfa, and blue-green algae supply minerals and reduce toxins. A high quality oil, such as hemp oil or Udo's Choice Oil Blend will provide the essential fatty acids necessary to heal and maintain many vital bodily processes.

If you are a non-smoker, you know how smoke clings to your hair and clothing for hours after you've been to a party or any smoke-filled place. Once you are home, shower, wash your hair, and change into smoke-free clothes. This is especially important in the evening so you don't sleep in smoke fumes all night. Smoky coats and clothing can be hung in the basement or laundry room or outdoors in a shed or verandah to air, before they go back into the closet. Or just wear something that can go right into the washing machine. If I know I am going somewhere smoky, I try to remember to take supplementary antioxidants (vitamins A, B complex, C, E, Co-Q10, zinc, kelp, and essential fatty acid oil) before and after the event.

If you smoke, regularly taking the supplemental antioxidants mentioned in this chapter may help protect you a little from some of the detrimental effects. A note to smokers who are interested in realistic help with quitting. Read Kathleen DesMaisons' book, *Potatoes not Prozac*, particularly the section entitled "Nicotine" in chapter 11. As with sugar, nicotine addiction is very much influenced by biochemistry and DesMaisons provides a multi-dimensional approach to help with this complex challenge.

98. HOUSEGUESTS.

Once you start enjoying a toxin-free life, one thing will get to you. Other people. You will notice who douses themselves with scent, fabric softener, and other chemicals, especially when they come into your wonderful, pollution-free house. One overnight visitor used such a powerful spray deodorant, my husband and I felt the toxic effects for a full week afterwards.

I now know the importance of asking guests to refrain from using such products in my house. Guests who are still in a masking state won't realize what they're doing to themselves (or others). You are fully within your rights to protect your toxin-free home and your family's health by asking guests or anyone who comes to work in your house for their cooperation. They don't intentionally endanger your health, or their own, but their lack of information is no reason you should suffer.

One friend even put up a small sign in the bathroom asking visitors not to use scented products and instead provides unscented shampoo, conditioner, and soap. This reminder helps guests who are groggy and forgetful in the morning not to make the mistake of following their regular scented routine. At the same time, they have the opportunity to try some of the excellent unscented products available.

When the weather is fine, guests can apply their chemically scented products outdoors (hairspray, perfume, aftershave, any spray product) or they can take the products along with them and apply them in a public restroom after leaving your house. If these seem like extreme measures, remember that what might be a minor inconvenience in a guest's morning could make a major difference to an entire week of your health, your mental and emotional functioning, and your ability to do your work, not to mention preventing unknown long-term effects. Your guests might even learn something from you!

Consider cotton thermal blankets or machine-washable cotton covers to protect your upholstered furniture from perfume-coated guests, or politely guide those guests to wooden chairs that can be sponged off if any scent clings to them. Be sure to hang scent-wearing guests' coats and scarves where they cannot directly touch yours, or you will have to clean perfume residues from your outdoor wear. When guests bring you scented gifts, smile sweetly and get the items out of your house as quickly as possible. Or, if you're feeling brave, tell them the truth—that you will not be able to use the gift—and give it back!

99. HAVE FUN. LOVE YOUR BODY FOR BEING THERE.

Most of this book focusses on ways to improve your health by working with aspects of your physical environment, but health is never a purely physical matter. Your health is very much affected by your thoughts, feelings, and spirit. As Candace Pert, Christiane Northrup, Hans Selye, Bernie Siegel, Dharma Khalsa, Wayne Dyer, Deepak Chopra, Joan Borysenko, and many, many other physicians and researchers have shown, stress, or *distress* as Hans Selye called it weakens the immune system, taxes the endocrine system, and wreaks general disaster on your body.

On the other hand, having fun, feeling good, thinking joyful thoughts, meditating, singing, dancing, playing, praying, laughing, and doing work you love create all kinds of positive physical, mental, and emotional effects. In fact, your attitude may be the most important aspect of your health.

Another important aspect of health is to appreciate your truly amazing body.

Our culture has a largely negative attitude towards the body, particularly if you're female. It's actually considered *normal* for women to criticize their bodies as much as possible, examining them for every flaw while comparing them to the current techno-fashion standard of beauty. Computer-enhanced photographs of ever-younger and increasingly anorexic models present bizarre images of "beauty" that are not only impossible to achieve, even by the models who pose for the pictures, but have little or no relation to reality.

And what is reality? Reality is that far more people are interested in living meaningful lives than in weighing 85 pounds. But we are all affected by the severe image-conciousness of our culture.

One way to separate yourself out from the self-conciousness and negativity this breeds is to stop focussing on what you fear is wrong with you. Thoughts and beliefs powerfully affect well-being. Practice gratitude towards your body. Thank your feet and legs for allowing you to walk, swim, dance or just get to the refrigerator. Appreciate your hands and the many actions they enable you to perform. Realize how wonderful it is to have teeth to chew your food with. Contemplate how amazing it is that your body knows how to keep your heart beating, regulate your temperature, digest your food, reproduce your skin and other cells, grow hair, circulate your blood, hear, taste, send neuropeptides to the right locations, maintain your kidney, liver, bladder and other organ functions, breathe, clear out toxins, and heal wounds, all without your conscious participation. All you really have to do to be healthy is to get out of your body's way, so it can function properly.

If you still find it difficult to appreciate the miracle of your physical body and all the amazing things it does for you, listen to Christopher Reeve's book-on-tape, *Still Me*.

And laugh. I believe laughter stimulates the immune system. As Dr. Bernie Siegel would no doubt say, they who laugh, last.

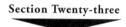

Top Ten

100. TOP TEN HOW TO STAY HEALTHY AND STILL EAT CHOCOLATE CHOICES.

1. Free your home from chemical toxins.

No one knows *all* the long term, cumulative effects of household chemicals on the human body, but the reports so far do not look good. Hormonal disruptions which affect the health and development of unborn children are one concern. Build-up of toxins in human tissue where they can become a contributing factor to disease is another.

To protect yourself and future generations of your family, clear all chemicals from your home, including *plastic bags and soft plastic containers, fabric softener, chlorine, detergent for laundry or dishes, harsh cleaners, drain cleaners, glues, polishes, room deodorants and air fresheners, oven cleaners, poisons, pesticides, solvents, gasoline, motor oil, and paints.* These chemicals are hazardous and must be disposed of at the toxic waste facility in your area. Call your local city or town hall for the location.

2. Free your body from toxic personal care products.

Personal care products contain chemicals which may endanger your health. Watch out for *hair dye, perfume, and antibacterial soaps*, and choose carefully when you select *deodorant, cosmetics, soaps, toothpaste, and feminine hygiene products.* If the products you're using contain synthetically-derived scent, petrochemicals or petrochemical derivatives, formaldehyde, mercury, bleach, fluoride, aluminum, lead or biocides, these are dangerous toxins which can build up in your body over time and contribute to life-threatening illnesses.

Old, unused medications and products containing alcohol (including any synthetically scented product), acetone (nail polish remover) or aerosol propellants (canned hairspray) *must* be disposed of at your local toxic waste facility.

3. Buy safe products.

One of the best ways you can protect yourself is to buy health-safe household and personal care products. There are many, many products made from natural source ingredients which will not endanger you.

You can clean your whole house with baking soda, borax, white vinegar or lemon juice, and liquid glycerin soap or a biodegradable all-purpose cleaning liquid. Not only is this cleaning kit cheaper than the usual collection of household cleaners, but it won't harm the environment, so while you're protecting your own health, you're also protecting the planet's. For laundry, use borax, laundry discs, and unscented, biodegradable laundry powder or liquid. Ecover, Nature Clean, Orange Apeel, and other companies make safe household cleaners and laundry products. The ingredients in safe products are usually revealed on the package so you know what you're buying.

Go for safe lawn and home renovation products, such as those available from Grassroots and Healthy Home Services, and buy natural bedding, clothing, and household linens. Favor glass, wood, and stainless steel in the kitchen over plastic. Do not use plastic cutting boards.

For personal care products, look at unscented, hypoallergenic or natural source lines such as Almay, Avalon Organics, Aveda All-Sensitive, Clinique, Ecco Bella, and Marcelle. Try hair care products from Aveda All-Sensitive, Avalon Organics, Infinity, Ferlow Brothers, Nature Clean, or Prairie Naturals. New plant-based, health-safe personal care products appear regularly, so scout your natural foods store and ask the staff what they recommend. Buy unbleached, unscented 100% cotton tampons and pads. Use non-fluoridated toothpaste; Tom's of Maine and Nature's Gate make good ones. Be cautious with personal care products that are antibacterial—they contain biocides which are toxins ('bio' means life and 'cide' means killer). Choose glycerin or vegetable-based unscented soaps or natural ingredient soaps scented with essential oils or herbs. Buy unscented sunscreen such as Ombrelle, and natural insect repellent made with citronella or tea tree oil.

4. Eat lots of vegetables.

Vegetables are like health insurance, only better. They give you anti-cancer, anti-pollution, pro-digestion advantages. The nutrients, fiber, and enzymes in vegetables keep your body functioning and healthy, enhance your digestion, and help clear out chemical toxins. Vegetables may well be the most important food group you can eat. Sam Graci recommends eating 10 servings per day!

5. Filter your water.

Ground water today is full of pollutants, even in wells in remote rural areas (because of farm run-off and bacteria). But water is so important to the healthy functioning of your body, it's absolutely vital to have top quality water for drinking, bathing, and cooking.

Source a good water filter and arrange for installation, or look for a company that delivers reverse-osmosis or distilled drinking water and arrange for delivery. Filtered drinking water is also available at many grocery stores. If your tap water is chlorinated and you buy bottled drinking water (rather than having a home filter system), install chlorine-removing shower heads in your bathrooms. These are available from environmental products stores and some hardware stores.

To avoid ingesting chemicals and pollutants, use filtered water to prepare hot beverages or juice made from concentrate, to wash raw vegetables and fruits, and to clean and cook any food that goes into your mouth. It's also a good idea to use filtered water for brushing your teeth.

6. Eat top quality oils.

Fats are used in many vital bodily processes including the regulation of heart rate, oxygen transfer, and brain function. To keep your brain and your physical health from degenerating, your diet needs to include the best quality fats and oils you can find. Overcooked, rancid, and solid fats and oils are a source of free-radicals which harm your body and contribute to disease and mental degeneration.

Go through your kitchen and throw out margarine and poor quality oils (all supermarket vegetable oils except extra virgin olive oil). Purchase extra virgin olive oil, organic hempseed oil, and/or organic butter. We also like Udo's Choice Oil Blend for its careful processing and essential fatty acid ratio. The best oils are sold in dark colored glass (not plastic) bottles to prevent light getting in and spoiling the oil. Organic butter will not contain the amounts of drug and/or chemical residue in conventional butter, lard, and margarine. If you can't eat butter, arrange your food choices to eliminate the need for a spreadable fat.

Use olive oil for salads, to mix with tuna or hard-boiled eggs for sandwiches, or to make your own mayonnaise. Hemp and Udo's Choice oils are highly nutritious—if you don't care for the taste on bread or vegetables, blend them into blender drinks where they won't be noticed. Don't cook with these two oils (they're destroyed by heat). Olive oil or butter can be used in small amounts in cooking. The healthiest way to cook with oil such as olive oil is to put a little water in the pan first to keep the oil from overheating.

Buy baked goods—breads, cookies, muffins—made with vegetable oil (safflower, sunflower, canola) rather than shortening or lard, or make your own with olive oil or organic butter.

7. Go sugar-free and eliminate white flour foods.

Sugar slows your immune function almost to a standstill, uses up nutrients you need for more important processes, rots your teeth, makes you fat, exhausts your adrenal glands, distorts your blood sugar and insulin levels, and disrupts your emotions and your thinking ability. White flour has many of the same effects on the body as sugar, as well as clogging up your intestines (remember making glue out of white flour and water in kindergarten?) Conventional flour is from wheat, one of the top allergens according to medical authorities. Infants do not develop the enzymes to digest grains before the age of six months to one year and can begin a life-long allergy when they're given flour products or formula containing some form of grain too early.

For sweeteners, switch to honey, stevia, rice syrup, barley malt, fruit juice concentrate or maple syrup. Buy bakery products, spreads (jams), and frozen desserts sweetened with any of these sugar alternatives and use them when making your own goodies. Or be really different and go completely sweet-free! Eat fruit for dessert. Instead of white flour products, buy whole grain baked goods, cereal, and flour. Try spelt, kamut, oat, quinoa, amaranth, and millet.

If you have a powerful sweet tooth that seems to run your life, look into literature on stabilizing blood sugar and stimulating brain chemicals in ways that are easy on your body, such as DesMaisons' *Potatoes Not Prozac* or Robertson's *Peak Performance Living*.

8. Eat organically raised food.

Organically raised food is more nutritious, tastes better, and is free of the chemical residues, radiation, hormones, drugs, and synthetic additives in conventionally grown foods.

Conventionally grown foods can *add* to your total toxic load, contributing to degenerative conditions. Organically raised foods are not only better for your body but for the planet, since they are grown by sustainable farming methods rather than agri-business methods which destroy land and pollute water with chemicals, drugs, and dangerous bacteria.

Since agricultural chemicals banned in North America are often sent to Third World nations, beware of conventionally grown crops imported from hot climates. The most polluted conventional crops from both North America and beyond are strawberries (strawberries that are not organically-grown have the highest levels of pesticides of any food!), bananas, apples, peaches, green and red peppers, especially from Mexico, canteloupe from Mexico, green beans, celery, pears, apricots, cucumbers, spinach, rice, oats, grapes from Chile, baby food, and soy products. Non-organic soy products are also heavily bio-engineered, which means they may be developed to contain pesticides, virus or genes from other species.

9. Spend some time in the sun every day.

For the last few years, we've been told time and time again that we have to protect our skin and eyes from the sun. We do need to protect ourselves from an *overdose* of rays by avoiding the sun at its peak hours during its peak seasons, but a moderate amount of sunlight is highly beneficial.

Spend some time outdoors every day, without sunglasses and preferably without prescription glasses, winter and summer. People who are lethargic and depressed in winter may also need full-spectrum lighting in the room(s) where they spend most of their time, to relieve symptoms of Seasonal Affective Disorder. Like plants, we need light.

If you are a committed sunglass-wearer, leave the glasses off for a few minutes each time you go outside, until your eyes re-adjust to natural light. Consult your physician first if you have a medical condition requiring protective lenses. Sunglasses were invented for pilots in World War II and are really only necessary in extreme conditions such as sparkling summer days on the water, bright sun on snowy ski slopes, or driving while facing into the setting sun. Continual wearing of sunglasses interferes with the eye's natural ability to adapt to changes in light and may be a factor in osteoporosis.

What are the benefits of going glasses-free outdoors? The full spectrum of sunlight assists in the creation of vitamin D, improves the uptake of calcium (strengthening bones), stimulates the immune system, helps to prevent Seasonal Affective Disorder, strengthens eyesight, and contributes to healthy skin, glands, and brain function. Since the body can't manufacture what sunlight provides or receive it from any other source, it is an *essential* ingredient to your health.

10. Relax, have fun, and laugh as often as possible. (And eat some really good chocolate!)

Ultimately, it's the *quality*, not the quantity, of your life and relationships (and chocolate) that matters most. Enjoy, and be healthy!

...AND FINALLY

If you are relatively healthy now, you may wonder why you should go to the trouble of following the suggestions in this book. Fear is one reason. I have read that fear is the strongest motivator of all the emotions. Certainly it is an emotion that starts many people on the road to better health, as it did me.

But after you begin, what is it that sustains you over the long term? I believe it is not fear, but love. Ultimately, it is the love of ourselves, our children, our parents, our friends, our pets, our homes, our communities, and of simply being alive that motivates us to create improvements. And the improvements we create individually ripple outward to improve life for everyone.

This beneficial ripple effect begins when you make a simple change like switching to a health-safe dish or laundry product. As your friends, and their friends, become interested and begin to make similar changes, everyone notices health improvements in themselves and their family members. At the same time, because fewer people are pouring toxic products into the water supply, a huge toxic burden begins to lift from the rivers and lakes. In this way, you help to create cleaner, safer water for yourself and for future generations. And when your water, air, home, and food are safe and toxin-free, you tend to have more energy available for your daily life and for the things you love to do. You may even find you have enough energy that you no longer need chocolate, coffee or treats to pump you up and keep you awake!

To me, the best reason to stay healthy is because it feels good, and feeling good is what life is all about.

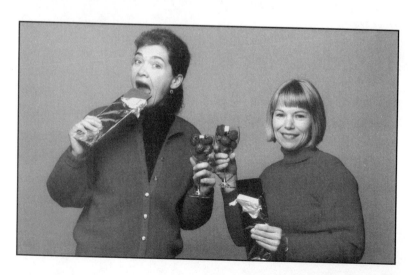

Chapter Notes

Chapter

7. Does perfume drive you wild?
- *contain chemicals*: Green, Nancy Sokol. *Poisoning Our Children*. Chicago, The Noble Press, 1991, pp. 90-1.
- *act as neurotoxins*: Dadd, Debra Lynn, *Nontoxic, Natural, & Earthwise*. Los Angeles: Jeremy P. Tarcher, Inc., 1996, pp. 302-3, and Rapp, Doris J., M.D. *The Impossible Child*. Buffalo, NY.: Practical Allergy Research Foundation, 1986.

8. Soap.
- *deodorant soaps*: Dadd., *op. cit.*, p. 212.
- *contain benzene*: Toronto Environmental Alliance, personal communication.

10. Hair care.
- *prematurely grey*: Kushi, Michio. *How to See Your Health: Book of Oriental Diagnosis*. Tokyo: Japan Publications, 1987, p. 108.
- *traditional herbal methods*: Hey, Barbara. *The Illustrated Book of Herbs*. London: New Holland, 1996, p. 171, and Mindell, Earl. *Earl Mindell's Herb Bible*. New York: Simon & Schuster/Fireside, 1992.

11. Deodorant.
- *deodorants don't work*: Panati, *Extraordinary Origins of Everyday Things*. New York: Perennial Library Harper & Row, 1987, pp. 254-6.

14. Cosmetics. Do you really have to suffer to be beautiful?
- *cosmetics in ancient times*: Panati, *op. cit.*, p. 224.
- *toxic beauty products*: Needleman, Herbert L., M.D., and Landrigan, Philip J., M.D. *Raising Children Toxic Free*. New York: Farrar, Straus, & Giroux, 1994, p. 11.
- *mutagens*: Colborn, Theo, and Dumanoski, Dianne, and Myers, John Peterson. *Our Stolen Future*. Dutton, 1996, p. 212.
- *Among these ingredients*: Dadd, *op. cit.*, and Green, *op. cit.*
- *affect her fetus*: Colborn, *op. cit.*, p. 212.

16. Sunscreen.
- *osteoporosis and osteomalacia*: Armstrong, Sally. "Veiled Threat." *Homemaker's Magazine*. Summer 1997.
- *plain sesame oil*: Erasmus, Udo. *Fats that Heal Fats that Kill*. Burnaby, B.C.: Alive Books, 1994.

17. Insect repellent.
- *oils that repel*: Hey, *op. cit.*, p. 160.
- *attracted to sweets*: Dufty, William. *Sugar Blues*. New York: Warner Books, 1993, p. 214.

18. Toothpaste and fluoride.
- *Calcium fluoride*: Dunne, Lavon J. *Nutrition Almanac, Third Edition*/Nutrition Search, Inc., John D. Kirschmann, director. New York: McGraw Hill, 1990, p. 72.
- *cavity-preventing effects*: Panati, *op. cit.*, p. 213.
- *more dangerous categories*: Dadd, *op. cit.*, p. 302, and Dunne, *op. cit.*, p. 73.
- *Down's syndrome*: Dunne, *ibid.*
- *preventing cavities*: Stay, Flora Parsa, D.D.S. *The Complete Book of Dental Remedies.* Garden City, NY.: Avery Publishing Group, 1996, p. 96.

19. Mercury amalgam fillings and metal in the mouth.
- *chronic health problems*: Balch, James F., M.D., and Balch, Phyllis A., C.N.C. *Prescription for Nutritional Healing.* Garden City Park, NY.: Avery Publishing Group, 1997, p. 386.

20. Feminine hygiene products.
- *formaldehyde, an irritant*: Rea, William J., M.D. *Chemical Sensitivity, volume 1.* Boca Raton, FL.: Lewis Publishers, 1992, *op. cit.*, p. 79.
- *toxic shock*: Dadd, *op. cit.*, p. 191.

21. Trouble in the laundry room.
- *mercury*: Balch, *op. cit.*, p. 386.

23. Natural fabric softener.
- *use herbs*: Hey, *op. cit.*, p. 114.
- *sponge the residue*: Oelrichs, Sherry. "Reducing Perfume Exposure." Information paper, 1985.

24. Stain removal without tears.
- *cancers of the gastrointestinal and urinary tracts*: Dadd, *op. cit.*, p. 300.
- *treatments for stains*: Dadd, *ibid.*, pp. 160-161, and "Recipes for Responsibility." *Stepping Lightly on the Earth.* Greenpeace Information Office, December 1995.

26. Additions to the medicine cabinet.
- *pneumococcal pneumonia*: Pomeranz, Bruce, M.D. *Alternative Medicine, A Clash of Paradigms.* Audiotape, November 29, 1991.
- *eliminating virus*: Erasmus, Udo. Lecture on healing properties of oils and essential fatty acids. Newmarket, October 8, 1998.

28. Frequent colds? Try this.
- *Sugars slow down*: Pizzorno, Joseph E. "POW! Supercharge Your Immune System." *Natural Health*, September/October 1994.

29. Trouble sleeping? Try this.
- *your brain replays*: Canfield, Jack. "Self Esteem and Peak Performance." Videotape.

30. Constipated? Try this.
- *every ten minutes*: Balch, *op. cit.*, p. 213.
- *flax seeds alleviate*: Erasmus, *op. cit.*, p. 285.

31. Menstrual discomfort? Try this.
- *levels of norepinephrine*: Robertson, Joel, M.D., with Monte, Tom. *Natural Prozac–Learning to Release Your Body's Own Antidepressants*. HarperSanFrancisco, 1997, p. 51.
- *"internal pollution"*: Erasmus, *op. cit.*, p. 350.

32. Make your home a pollution-free oasis.
- *cancer in women*: Green, *op. cit.*, p. 87.
- *chemical compounds*: Rea, *op. cit.*, p. 19.
- *adolescent delinquency*: Hatherill, J. Robert, Ph.D. "Are violent teens more toxic?" *Lifelines*, September & October 1999, pp. 1 & 8.
- *Agent Orange*: Erasmus, *op. cit.*

33. Are your cleaners safe?
- *Chlorine...birth defects*: Dadd, *op. cit.*, pp. 298-305.

36. Contain your plastic bags.
- *Some plastics*: Dadd, *op. cit.*, p. 305, and *Living Safety Magazine*, Spring 1996, pp. 8-10.

39. Super-sealed houses.
- *can't escape*: "Are Chemicals In Your Home Making You Sick?" *Toronto Star*, December 4, 1993, p. L10.
- *use plants*: "Houseplants: Fresh Air Factories." *Alive*, January 1998, p. 80, and Wolverton, B.C. "How To Grow Fresh Air." *Country Living's Healthy Living*, February/March 1998, pp. 86-87.

40. The trouble with mold.
- *mold with asthma*: Mandell, Marshall, M.D., and Scanlon, Lynne Waller. *Dr. Mandell's 5-Day Allergy Relief System*. New York: Pocket Books, 1980, pp. 228-9.
- *depression...tiredness*: Rapp, *op. cit.*, p. 99.
- *molds and fungus*: Constantini, A.V., M.D., "Fungal/Mycotoxins in Human Health." Fungal Toxins Conference, Toronto, October 1, 1994.
- *10 million micro-organisms*: "Experts Probe 'Mould' In Houses." *Toronto Star*, March 13, 1994, p. L5.

41. About scent.
- *pounds of flower petals*: Panati, Charles, *op. cit.*, p. 240.

42. Keep paint, glue and solvents out of your indoor air.
- *Johns Hopkins*, Dadd, *op. cit.*, p. 274.

43. Natural Gas.
- *Gas stoves*: Ferrie, Helke. "Stop Cooking with Gas!" *Alive Magazine*, December 1997, p. 49.
- *Nitrogen dioxide*: Ferrie, *ibid.*, p. 49.

47. Healthy fabrics for interiors.
- *Fabric dyes*: Kapner, Elizabeth M. in Dickey, Lawrence, M.D., ed. *Clinical Ecology*. Springfield, Illinois: Charles C. Thomas, 1976, p. 356.

50. Electromagnetic frequencies.
- *60 hertz*: Dadd, *op. cit.*, p. 59.
- *300 hertz*: Needleman, *op. cit.*, p. 154.

51. Take poisons seriously.
- *three variations*: Needleman, *ibid.*, p. 115.
- *2,000 "so-called" inert*: Dadd, *op. cit.*, p. 304.
- *formaldehyde, asbestos*: Green, *op. cit.*, p. 48.
- *crop losses*: Benyus, Janine M. *Biomimicry*. New York: William Morrow and Company, 1997, p. 18.
- *DDT*: Colborn, *op. cit.*, p. 138.
- *acre for acre*: Dadd, *op. cit.*, p. 163.
- *hormone disruptors*: Colborn, *op. cit.*, pp. 203-4.
- *estrogenic effects*: Weil, Andrew, M.D. *8 Weeks to Optimum Health*. New York: Alfred Knopf, 1997, pp. 85-6.

54. Choosing fertilizers and lawn care companies.
- *Agent Orange*: Colborn, *op. cit.*, pp. 113-4.
- *most toxic synthetic*: Needleman, *op. cit.*, p. 118.
- *Diazinon*: Needleman, *ibid.*, p. 125.
- *Dioxin contains carbon*: Toronto Environmental Alliance, personal communication.

55. Lawn alternatives.
- *In the midwest*: Benyus, *op. cit.*, pp. 15-16.

58. Drink water.
- *less than a week*: Dunne, *op. cit.*, p. 93.
- *Lack of adequate*: Batmanghelidj, F., M.D., *Your Body's Many Cries for Water*. Falls Church, VA.: Global Health Solutions, 1996, p. 18.

59. Improve your water.
- *frozen in glaciers*: Dunne, *op. cit.*, p. 92.
- *raw sewage*: Leckie, Stephen. "Why Environmentalists Should Be Vegetarian." Toronto Vegetarian Association information paper, June 18, 1993.
- *one beef cow*: "Recipe for a Cow." *Lifelines*, July & August 1994, p. 11.
- *Lead can accumulate*: Needleman, *op. cit.*, p. 77.
- *removed by boiling*: Green, *op. cit.*, p. 151.

61. Eat for nutrient value.
- *top food allergens*: Rapp, *op. cit.*, pp. 4 & 44, and Berger, Stuart M., M.D. *What Your Doctor Didn't Learn in Medical School.* New York: Avon Books, 1989, pp. 277, 278 & 280.

62. Eat something different every day.
- *developing food sensitivities*: Mandell, *op. cit.*, p. 36.
- *four or five days*: Philpott, Nielsen & Pearson in Dickey, *op. cit.*, p. 473.

64. Take enzymes.
- *as you get older*: Balch and Balch, *op. cit.*, p. 48, and Erasmus, Udo, Ph.D. "Adding Spark to Your Life", *Alive*, November 1998, p. 52.
- *both pancreatic enzymes*: Keith, David R. "Enzymes: The Missing Link." *Alive*, November 1998, p. 15.

65. Be careful with moldy and yeasty foods.
- *health problems including*: Fungal Toxins Conference, Toronto, October 1, 1994.

66. Buy organically-grown or at least avoid the most chemically-polluted crops.
- *number one polluting*: Benyus, *op. cit.*, p. 19.
- *watch out for*: Weil, *op. cit.*, p. 84, and Stephens, Francine and Lydon, Betsy. "10 Must-Eat Organic Foods." *Utne Reader*, January-February 1998, pp. 78-9.

69. What happens when your body clears out toxins? About detoxing.
- *jumping on a trampoline*: Kenton, Leslie. *Cellulite Revolution.* London, England: Ebury Press, 1994, p. 59.

72. Snack ideas.
- *aflatoxin, a fungal carcinogen*: Galapeaux, Edward A. in Dickey, *op. cit.*, p. 403.

73. Protein.
- *Great Lakes fish*: Colborn, *op. cit.*, pp. 190-4.
- *Milk and meat*: Redvers, Rick. "Don't Have A Cow!" *Lifelines*, May & June 1996, pp. 1 & 6.
- *a little oil*: Erasmus lecture.

74. Eat only the best oils.
- *brains are 60%*: Erasmus lecture.
- *blamed on fats*: Erasmus, *ibid.*

75. Fats and oils: which is better? Refined, or less polished but more sincere?
For more information on fats and oils, their processing and health consequences, read Erasmus, Udo. *Fats that Heal Fats that Kill.* Burnaby, B.C.: Alive Books, 1994.

77. Is it better to be vegetarian?
- *vegetarianism works best*: Colbin, *Food and Healing*, New York: Ballantine Books, 1996, p. 121.

- *is not convinced*: Klaper, Michael, M.D. "The 'Blood Type Diet'–Fact or Fiction?" *Lifelines*, January & February 1999, pp. 1 & 6.

78. *Eat more vegetables.*
- *dark leafy greens*: Colbin, *op. cit.*, p. 199.

79. *Why is calcium such a big deal and how much is enough?*
- *Calcium helps form*: Balch, *op. cit.*, p. 23, and Dunne, *op. cit.*, pp. 66-7.

80. *It's not how much calcium you eat, it's how much you absorb or lose.*
- *full body veils*: Armstrong, *op. cit.*, p. 28.
- *uses the sunlight*: Balch, *op. cit.*, p. 19, and Nutrition Action Newsletter, volume 25, #3, April 1998, p. 7.
- *return to homeostasis*: Appleton, Nancy. *Healthy Bones.* Garden City Park, NY.: Avery Publishing Group, 1991.
- *people with osteoporosis*: Colbin, *op. cit.*, p. 161.

81. *What about dairy?*
- *Cow's milk is higher*: Colbin, *op. cit.*, p. 150-1.
- *sulfur amino acids*: Schiller, Dave. "Calcium Controversy." *Lifelines*, July & August 1996, p.9.
- *mucus-forming*: This is why professional singers often avoid dairy products. They can't afford to cough in the middle of a solo.

87. *Sugar, vampire of the food world.*
- *The chemicals include:* Lake, Rhody. "Get The Sugar Out–And The Fat In!" *Alive*, November 1997, p. 76.

88. *But I brush my teeth so why shouldn't I eat sugar?*
- *inhibits your immune*: Pizzorno, *op. cit.*, p. 126.
- *German researchers*: Lake, Rhody, *op. cit.*
- *hyperactivity, lack of:* Colbin, *op. cit.*, p. 190
- *genetic narrowing*: Colbin, *ibid.*

91. *Aim for sweet-freedom.*
- *25% of what most people eat*: Khalsa, Dharma Singh, M.D. *Brain Longevity.* New York: Warner Books, 1997.
- *strict vegetarians who*: Colbin, *op. cit.*, p. 119.
- *Hitler, a vegetarian*: Colbin, *ibid.*, p. 120.

97. *Smoking.*
- *about 4,000 chemicals*: Balch, *op. cit.*, pp. 485-6.
- *substances in cigarettes*: Balch, *ibid.*, and Dunne, *op. cit.*, p. 162.
- *Vitamin supplementation*: Balch, *op. cit.*, p. 486.
- *excess cadmium damages*: Dunne, *op. cit.*, p. 66.

References

Abrams, Karl J. *Algae to the Rescue!* Studio City, CA.: Logan House Publications, 1996.

Appleton, Nancy. *Healthy Bones.* Garden City Park, NY.: Avery Publishing Group, 1991.

"Are Chemicals In Your Home Making You Sick?" *Toronto Star*, December 4, 1993.

Armstrong, Sally. "Veiled Threat." *Homemaker's Magazine.* Summer 1997.

Balch, James F., M.D., and Balch, Phyllis A., C.N.C. *Prescription for Nutritional Healing.* Garden City Park, NY.: Avery Publishing Group, 1997.

Balch, James F., M.D., *10 Natural Remedies that can Save Your Life.* New York, NY.: Doubleday, 1999.

Batmanghelidj, F., M.D., *Your Body's Many Cries for Water.* Falls Church, VA.: Global Health Solutions, 1996.

Benyus, Janine M. *Biomimicry.* New York: William Morrow and Company, 1997.

Berger, Stuart M., M.D. *What Your Doctor Didn't Learn in Medical School.* New York: Avon Books, 1989.

Bland, Jeffery. *Digestive Enzymes.* New Canaan, CT.: Keats Publishing, 1983.

Canfield, Jack. "Self Esteem and Peak Performance." Videotape.

Colbin, Annemarie. *Food and Healing.* New York: Ballantine Books, 1996.

Colborn, Theo, and Dumanoski, Dianne, and Myers, John Peterson. *Our Stolen Future.* Dutton, 1996.

Constantini, A.V., M.D. "Fungal/Mycotoxins in Human Health." Fungal Toxins Conference, Toronto, October 1, 1994.

Dadd, Debra Lynn. *Nontoxic, Natural, & Earthwise.* Los Angeles: Jeremy P. Tarcher, Inc., 1996.

DesMaisons, Kathleen. *Potatoes not Prozac.* New York: Simon & Schuster, 1998.

"Despair Affects Artery Health." *Toronto Star*, September 20, 1997.

"Desperately Seeking Vegetables." *Toronto Star,* June 24, 1992.

"Diatomaceous Earth." *Earthly*goods information paper.

Dickey, Lawrence D., M.D., ed. *Clinical Ecology.* Springfield, Illinois: Charles C. Thomas, 1976.

Dufty, William. *Sugar Blues.* New York: Warner Books, 1993.

Dunne, Lavon J. *Nutrition Almanac, Third Edition*/Nutrition Search, Inc., John D. Kirschmann, director. New York: McGraw Hill, 1990.

Erasmus, Udo. *Fats that Heal Fats that Kill.* Burnaby, B.C.: Alive Books, 1994.

Erasmus, Udo. Lecture on healing properties of oils and essential fatty acids. Newmarket, October 8, 1998.

"Experts Probe 'Mould' In Houses." *Toronto Star*, March 13, 1994.

Ferrie, Helke. "Stop Cooking with Gas!" *Alive/the Green Magazine*, December 1997.

Fulder, Stephen. *The Ginger Book.* Garden City, N.Y.: Avery Publishing Group, 1996.

Gemmer, Erwin, M.D. *Who Stole America's Health?* Audiotape, February 1996.

Gottschall, Elaine. *Food and the Gut Reaction.* Kirkton, ON.: The Kirkton Press, 1986.

Graci, Sam with Diamond, Harvey. *The Power of Superfoods.* Scarborough, ON.: Prentice Hall, 1997.

Green, Nancy Sokol. *Poisoning Our Children.* Chicago: The Noble Press, 1991.

Hatherill, J. Robert. "Are violent teens more toxic?" *Lifelines,* September & October 1999.

"Heinz to start organic food division." *National Post,* February 10, 2000.

Hey, Barbara. *The Illustrated Book of Herbs.* London: New Holland, 1996.

"Houseplants: Fresh Air Factories." *Alive,* January 1998.

Huggins, Hal A., D.D.S. *It's All In Your Head.* Garden City Park, NY.: Avery Publishing Group, 1993.

Keith, David R. "Enzymes: The Missing Link." *Alive,* November 1998.

Kenton, Leslie. *Cellulite Revolution.* London: Ebury Press, 1994.

Khalsa, Dharma Singh, M.D. *Brain Longevity.* New York: Warner Books, 1997.

Klaper, Michael, M.D. "The "Blood Type Diet"–Fact or Fiction?" *Lifelines,* January & February 1999.

Kushi, Michio. *A Natural Approach to Allergies.* New York: Japan Publications, 1985.

Kushi, Michio. *How to See Your Health: Book of Oriental Diagnosis.* Tokyo: Japan Publications, 1987.

Lake, Rhody. "Get The Sugar Out–And The Fat In!" *Alive,* November 1997.

Leckie, Stephen. "Cow's Milk." Toronto Vegetarian Association information paper, June 1, 1993.

Leckie, Stephen. "Why Environmentalists Should Be Vegetarian." Toronto Vegetarian Association information paper, June 18, 1993.

Lee, John R., M.D. *What Your Doctor May Not Tell You About Menopause.* New York: Warner, 1996.

Liberman, Jacob, O.D. *Take Off Your Glasses and See.* New York: Crown, 1995.

Living Safety Magazine, Spring 1996.

Mandell, Marshall, M.D., and Scanlon, Lynne Waller. *Dr. Mandell's 5-Day Allergy Relief System.* New York: Pocket Books, 1980.

Mindell, Earl. *Earl Mindell's Herb Bible.* New York: Simon & Schuster/Fireside, 1992.

Mittelstaedt, Martin. "Environmental Factors Blamed For Higher Cancer Rates." *Globe & Mail,* March 27, 1999.

Moyers, Bill. *Healing and the Mind.* New York: Doubleday, 1993.

Needleman, Herbert L., M.D., and Landrigan, Philip J., M.D. *Raising Children Toxic Free.* New York: Farrar, Straus, & Giroux, 1994.

Northrup, Christiane, M.D. *Women's Bodies, Women's Wisdom.* New York: Bantam Books, 1994.

Ohrbach, Barbara Milo. *The Scented Room.* New York: Clarkson N. Potter, 1986.

Oelrichs, Sherry. "Reducing Perfume Exposure." Information paper, 1985.

Ornish, Dean, M.D. *Love and Survival: The Scientific Basis for the Healing Power of Intimacy.* New York: Harper Collins, 1998.

Padus, Emrika et al. *The Complete Guide to Your Emotions and Your Health.* Emmaus, PA.: Rodale Press, 1992.

Panati, Charles. *Extraordinary Origins of Everyday Things.* New York: Perennial Library Harper & Row, 1987.

Pert, Candace, Ph.D. *Molecules of Emotion.* New York: Scribner, 1997.

Philpott, William H., M.D., and Kalita, Dwight K., M.D. *Brain Allergies–The Psycho Nutrient Connection.* New Canaan, CT.: Keats Publishing, 1986.

Pizzorno, Joseph E. "POW! Supercharge Your Immune System." *Natural Health*, September/October 1994.

"Pollutants Affect Behavior: Researchers." *Toronto Star*, November 2, 1996.

Pomeranz, Bruce, M.D. *Alternative Medicine, A Clash of Paradigms.* Lecture, November 29, 1991.

Randolph, Theron G., M.D., and Moss, Ralph W. *An Alternative Approach to Allergies.* New York: Bantam Book, 1982.

Rapp, Doris J., M.D. *The Impossible Child.* Buffalo, NY.: Practical Allergy Research Foundation, 1986.

Rea, William J., M.D. *Chemical Sensitivity, volume 1.* Boca Raton, FL.: Lewis Publishers, 1992.

"Recipes for Responsibility." *Stepping Lightly on the Earth.* Greenpeace Information Office, December 1995.

Redvers, Rick. "Don't Have A Cow!" *Lifelines*, May & June 1996.

Robertson, Joel, M.D., with Monte, Tom. *Natural Prozac–Learning to Release Your Body's Own Antidepressants.* HarperSanFrancisco, 1997.

Rowland, David. *The Nutritional Bypass.* Parry Sound, ON.: Health Naturally Publications, 1995.

Russell, Dick. "Is Your House Making You Sick?" *Natural Health*, March/April 1994: 80-83.

Sarick, Lila. "To Spray Or Not To Spray?–That Is The Question." *Globe and Mail*, August 29, 1998.

Schiller, Dave. "Calcium Controversy." *Lifelines*, July & August 1996.

Schneider, Meir and Larkin, Maureen. *The Handbook of Self-Healing.* London: Penguin Arkana, 1994.

"Should You Use A Water Filter?" *Consumer Reports*, July 1997.

Stay, Flora Parsa, D.D.S. *The Complete Book of Dental Remedies.* Garden City, NY.: Avery Publishing Group, 1996.

Stephens, Francine and Lydon, Betsy. "10 Must-Eat Organic Foods." *Utne Reader*, January-February 1998.

Thorne, Stephen. "MDs Say Carpets Responsible For More And More Illnesses." *Toronto Star*, December 3, 1994.

Wallich, Joel, M.D. "Dead Doctors Don't Lie." Audiotape.

Weed, Susun. *Menopausal Years The Wise Woman Way.* Woodstock, NY: Ash Tree Publishing, 1992.

Weil, Andrew, M.D. *8 Weeks to Optimum Health.* New York: Alfred Knopf, 1997.

Weil, Andrew, M.D. *Spontaneous Healing.* New York: Alfred Knopf, 1995.

Wolverton, B.C. "How To Grow Fresh Air." *Country Living's Healthy Living*, February/March 1998.

Wolverton, B.C. *How to Grow Fresh Air.* Viking Penguin, 1996.

Zamm, Alfred V., M.D., with Gannon, Robert. *Why Your House May Endanger Your Health.* New York: Touchstone, 1982.

Resource Guide, Cookbooks and Useful Books

Code:
EPS = environmental product stores
NFS = natural foods stores
GS = grocery stores: some grocers, such as Zehr's, Loblaws, & Dominion have large natural products sections.
GEP = Grassroots Environmental Products
GAI = Gaiam , a lifestyle company
HHS = Healthy Home Services

This guide is in alphabetical order according to name or type of product or service. Fresh food products such as oils and breads contain no preservatives and must be kept in the fridge or freezer.

The products listed are examples of what is available in the marketplace. While you can mail-order them from almost anywhere, we also urge you to seek out health-supporting products developed and manufactured in your local area. The farther a product has to be shipped, the more packaging and polluting transportion it requires, adding to your personal toxic load as well as that of the larger environment. Easy-to-locate brands such as Clinique are not listed here.

Also check the web, whether or not an address is listed here. Listings may have changed without notice.

Acidophilus
At NFS, usually in capsule form, usually refrigerated.

Air Cleaners, Heat Recovery Ventilators & Clean Air Furnaces
1. Bionaire (portable air cleaners), www.bionaire.com, 1-800-561-6478
2. Lifebreath by NuTech Energy Systems: www.lifebreath.com, 1-800-494-4185
3. GAI, GEP, HHS

Arnica Montana
At NFS, herbal stores & some pharmacies, in drops (tincture) or tablets.

Avalon Organics
At NFS or www.avalonnaturalproducts.com

Baby Care Products
At EPS, some NFS, and by mail order from GAI, HHS, and Beebalm & Basil (see listing below).

Baking Soda
Available in bulk at NFS & EPS. Also Loblaws' cleaning products aisle in 3 kg. boxes. Mail order from GEP or HHS.

Baking Paper
1) Baker's Mate non-stick Parchment Paper, at GS & cooking speciality stores.
2) "If you care" unbleached baking paper, at NFS, EPS, or contact Anke Kruse Organics 519-853-3899.

Beebalm and Basil: Herb-based personal care products, baby care, pet care, teas, insect repellent & sunscreen
View & order through www.webruler.com/beebalm or phone 613-731-1296 or 1-877-524-4705.

Borax
In cleaning product section of NFS, EPS & GS. Bulk or mail order from GEP and HHS.

Buckwheat Husk Pillows
At bedding shops, Oriental stores, or call 416-763-0949

Burt's Bees, Inc.: insect repellent, lip gloss, anti-poison ivy soap, facial in a kit, gardener's kit–also good for hikers & other outdoor types
Raleigh, NC 27612, 1-800-849-7112, www.burtsbees.com or buy at EPS & some NFS. Also at GEP.

Cardboard Storage Boxes
At stationery & department stores, & IKEA.

Carob Rocky Choc
At NFS, or contact: Sunfresh Organics, 2155 Leanne Blvd., Mississauga, Ontario. 905-855-1957.

Cellulose Bags
Order from GAI or from French's Paper (Hamilton) 905-574-0275.

Chocolate-Organic & Sugar-free
At NFS, or contact:
1. La Siembra Co-operative Inc., 1325 Essex St., Ottawa, ON K1H 7P1, www.lasiembra.com
(Fair Trade Organic Cocoa Powder)
2. Rapunzel Pure Organics, 122 Smith Road, Kinderhook, NY 12106. 1-800-207-2814, www.rapunzel.com
(Rapunzel Pure Organic Cocoa Powder - Unsweetened)
3. Sunspire, 2114 Adams Avenue, San Leandro, CA 94577. 510-569-9731.
(Sunspire Grain Sweetened Chocolate Chips - sweetened with malted barley and corn. Not organic.)

Chocolate, Bars & Gift Boxes-Organic, sweetened with Organic Sugar
At NFS, or contact:
1. Hawaiian Vintage Chocolate, www.hawaiianchocolate.com, 808-735-8494
2. Pronatec Swiss Chocolate, www.pronatec.com
3. Terra Nostra by KFM Foods International Inc., P.O. Box 71054, Vancouver, B.C., V6N 4J9, email: info@venussweets.com, www.venussweets.com, fax: 604-267-3582

Coffee Substitute
1. Raja's Cup, grain-free, antioxidant-rich: at NFS or call 1-800-255-8332
2. Stand up. Start snapping your fingers with both hands, repeatedly. Now stamp your feet. Keep snapping and stamping faster and faster and breath *deeply*. Stop when you feel really energized.

Condoms, Non-Petrochemical
Trojan Kling Tite, Naturalamb Non-latex condoms, at pharmacies. Not for the prevention of STDs.

Cosmetics, Natural
Ecco Bella: at NFS or www.eccobella.com

Cotton Bed Linens: 100% Unbleached Cotton
For catalogue, write to: Clothes & Friendly, P.O. Box 23074, Ottawa, Ontario K2A 4E2
Also by mail order from GAI (bedding, nightwear, shower curtains) or HHS (organic cotton bedding)

Cotton Thermal Blankets
At department and bedding stores or by mail order from GAI.

Crystal Aire and Crystal Shield
Order from Smith's Pharmacy, 416-488-2600 or from www.greenhome.com

Deodorants & Deodorant Stones
At NFS, EPS, GAI and some natural cosmetics stores.

Diatomacheous Earth
At EPS, or mail order from GEP.

Drain Cleaner
EPS, GAI, HHS

Dry Cleaning & professional Wetcleaning
Dry: www.greenearthcleaning.com
Wet: www.greenhome.com, see home page

Ecover Cleaning Products
At GS, NFS, EPS. Or contact: ECOVER Inc., P.O. Box 5145, Huntington Beach, CA 92615

Enamel Buckets with Lids
At kitchen speciality stores & hardware stores.

Enzymes/Digestive Enzymes/Udo's Choice Enzymes/Ultrazyme
At NFS. Or contact Flora Inc. for Udo's (see below) Also see Wobenzym listing.

Feminine Hygiene Products
At NFS, EPS, HHS, & www.greenhome.com. Or contact:
1. Organic Essentials, Rt. 1 Box 120, O'Donnell, TX 79351, 1-800-765-6491.
2. Eco*fem* tampons and pads, made by Rogg AG, Germany. Distributed by Eco*fem* Products, Canada, 6872 Barrisdale Drive, Mississauga, Ontario L5N 2H4.
3. Eco Yarn Co. tampons, 249A Darlinghurst Road, Darlinghurst, NSW 2010 Australia. Distributed by Eco Yarn Canada, Harding POB 32227, Richmond Hill, Ontario L4C 9S3, 416-410-9015.
4. Natracare tampons and pads, BodyWise (UK) Limited, Bristol BS12 4DX, England. In North America: 191 University Blvd., Suite 219, Denver, CO 80206.

Flea Shampoo, Natural: see Pet Care, below

Flora Inc.
Products at NFS or contact at: Box 73, Lynden WA 98264, 1-800-446-2110, www.florainc.com
In Canada: 1-888-436-6697, www.florahealth.com

Food Sensitivity Testing
For practitioners in your area, contact:
1. American Academy of Environmental Medicine, phone 316-684-5500, www.aaem.com
2. International Association of Specialized Kinesiologists, Box 415, Bristol, VT, USA 05443, Fax: 802-453-6197
3. Canadian Association of Specialized Kinesiology, Box 74508 Kitsilano Postal Unit, Vancouver, B.C., V6K 4P4, phone: 604-669-8481, fax: 604-669-8099.
4. check your local natural health publications or directory of wellness practitioners

Full Spectrum Lightbulbs
At EPS, some NFS. GAI, GEP, HHS.

Fun: Adventures in Nature! Canoeing, Backpacking, Custom Trips, Artists Workshop, Adventures for All, Women Only, Men Only, Vegetarian Option
Contact Windsong Adventures: 905-826-7408 or www.windsongadventures.com. Also, see GAI Travel.

Furniture
Healthy Everything, 212-896-8440, www.healthyeverything.com. Also GAI.

Furniture Polish
At EPS, HHS, www.greenhome.com, & household products stores or write:
Natural Beeswax Furniture Polish, 34-36 McLachlan Avenue, Rushcutter's Bay NSW 2011
Australia, phone (02) 9332-4455

Ginger Root Capsules
At NFS, herbal stores & some pharmacies.

Glycerin Soap
At NFS, EPS, some GS & country stores.

Greens+
At NFS, some pharmacies, & Sears health & fitness shops. www.greensplus.com

GAI - *Gaiam, a lifestyle company:* Extensive product listing including household cleaners
and cleaning tools, personal care, furniture, air & water filters, natural deodorizers, cotton
dress & shoe bags, cellulose bags, hemp shower curtains, household linens, clothing,
exercise options, books, videos and pest control. Also travel & zine. www.gaiam.com

GEP - *Grassroots Environmental Products:* Over 2,000 products including Nature Clean,
household cleaners, energy-efficient products, air & water filters, household linens,
personal care products, feminine hygiene products, clothing, books, office supplies, &
home accessories (candles, etc.) Retail & international mail order. 372 Danforth Avenue,
Toronto, Canada. phone 416-466-2841, e-mail: grassroots@web.net

HHS - *Healthy Home Services:* Unique range of health-safe products including household
cleaners, laundry & dish cleaners, personal care, baby care, natural pet line, organic
bedding, home renovation & repair, garden & lawn, air & water filters, pest control, green
gifts for kids, this book. Services: Chemical-free Lawn Care, Healthy Home Assessment.
www.healthyhomeservices.ca, phone 1-866-870-6970 or 416-410-4247 or by fax
905-882-1747

Hemp Products
- Hempoline: organic hemp clothing, accessories, bags, soap, coffee filters. Mail order:
phone or fax: 613-969-0754, www.canada-shops.com/stores/werfamily
- Hempola Valley Farms. To order pancake mix, flour, food, oils, soap, massage oil:
www.hempola.com
- Nutiva Shelled Hempseed: NFS or 1-800-993-HEMP, www.nutiva.com

Herbs, non-irradiated
"Frontier Herbs" or "Spice Garden" at NFS and herbalists. Herb mixtures from Beebalm &
Basil.

Home Environment Testing
1. Contact HHS for the Healthy Home Assessment
2. Centre for Home Environment Testing, 1-888-633-1690 or 905-726-1689 (GTA, Barrie, Hamilton, & Ottawa)

Honey & Nut Snack Bars (peanut-free & organic)
At NFS, or have your retailer order from Honey Bar, 1-800-851-7776, or Anke Kruse Organics Inc. 519-853-3899, fax 519-853-5155.

Infinity Shampoo & Conditioner
At NFS, GEP, or contact:
Infinity Herbal Products, Division of Jedmon Products Ltd., 333 Rimrock, Toronto, Ontario M3J 3J9, 416-631-4000

Insect Repellent
At NFS, EPS, GAI, GEP, & HHS, Beebalm & Basil, Burt's Bees, or: Thursday Plantation Laboratories Ltd., Pacific Highway, Ballina 2478 Australia, www.thursdayplantation.com

Kydophilus
At NFS, in supplements section.

Laminate flooring
Made by Pergo, Mannington, etc. Sold at hardware/home renovation materials stores.

Laundry Detergent, Scent-free (conventional)
President's Choice (PC) Ultra Laundry Detergent Unscented. In U.S. at Harris-Teeter & Jewel. In Canada at Loblaws & No-Name.

Laundry Discs
At NFS, EPS, GEP, or from: Teldon Ltd., 1-800-663-2212

Lip Gloss/Balm
Webber Vitamin E for Lips, Karitea Natural Lip Balm, Unpetroleum lip balm, Burt's Bees at NFS, EPS, GEP.

Marcelle Products
At pharmacy cosmetic counters.

Meat, Additive-Free: Cumbrae Farms, Rowe Farms
At NFS, some butcher shops, or have your butcher or NFS contact Cumbrae Farms 519-587-5856 or Rowe Farms, or any local farmer who produces poultry & meat naturally (with good quality feed & without hormones & antibiotics).
In England, contact Heritage Prime at Shedbush Farm 01297 489304.
HeritagePrime@aol.com

Milk Thistle
At NFS, in capsules or tincture, in supplements section.

Mouth Wash
The Natural Dentist Herbal Mouth and Gum Therapy, at NFS, Supplements Plus, or contact Woodstock Natural Products, 1-800-827-5617.

Natural Vision Improvement
In North America: www.visioneducators.org
In Europe: www.seeing.org

Nature's Blends
Organic, petrochemical-free hair products scented with botanical essesnces. At NFS or call 1-888-265-2615.

Nature Clean
Unscented, biodegradable household cleaners, laundry & personal care products. At NFS, EPS, some GS, GEP, HHS, www.greenhome.com, or Walmarts with nutritional centers (Canada only). www.franktross.com, Frank T. Ross & Sons Ltd., 6550 Lawrence Avenue East, Scarborough, ON, Canada M1C 4A7, 416-282-1107

Olbas Oil & Throat Pastilles
At NFS & some pharmacies or contact Flora.

Ombrelle (scent-free) Sunscreen Lotion
At pharmacies.

Orange aPEEL
Citrus-based all purpose cleaning concentrate. Also neutralizes skunk smell. Safe for pets. 1-800-956-6866, www.orangeapeel.com

Organic Foods
At NFS, GAI, GS such as Loblaws, Dominion, Costco and Zehrs, local organic home delivery services, some farmer's markets and pick-your-own farms. Also, in the US, order from Diamond Organics, 1-888-Organic, www.diamondorganics.com

Organic Country Shampoo & Conditioner
At NFS & some pharmacies, or have your retailer contact: Anke Kruse Organics Inc. 519-853-3899, fax 519-853-5155.

Organic Lawn Services
Check ads in your health publications or phone local environmental association. Contact HHS for organic lawn products.

Paint
HHS, GAI, www.greenhome.com, and Miller Paint Co., 503-255-0190,
www.millerpaint.com

Pet Care, Natural: Paw Rescue, Sunscreen, Flea Repellent, Invisible Boot, Herbal Shampoo
At some NFS and EPS. HHS, GAI, and Beebalm & Basil.

Pet Food, Natural
At NFS and some pet food stores, e.g. Global.

Protein Powders-dairy & egg free
At NFS. Or contact:
1. NutriBiotic, Lakeport, CA 95453, 707-263-0411, for organic rice protein powder
2. Swiss Herbal Remedies Ltd., Richmond Hill, ON L4B 4C2, 905-886-9500, for soy
protein powder

Pure Synergy
At some NFS. Or write The Synergy Company, HC 64 Box 2901, Castle Valley, Utah
84532-9613, 1-800-338-6138, www.synergy-co.com. Or from www.diamondorganics.com

Quinoa cereals, Ancient Harvest
At NFS. Or contact: Quinoa Corporation, P.O. Box 1039, Torrance, CA 90505

RayAway
P.O. Box 746387, Arvada, Colorado 80006, www.rayaway.com or contact: Healers Who
Share, Box 76, Stettler, Alberta T0C 2L0, 403-742-2863, fax 403-742-4507. In Toronto,
order from Markie Pharmacy, 416-969-9332

Rescue Remedy
A Bach flower remedy, at NFS, herbalists, & some pharmacies.

Rubber Totes Bags, Backpacks, Wallets and Garment Bags
Contact: Gentis International 416-487-4118, or gentis@better.net

Rugs &/or non-slip rug holds:
GAI, IKEA, www.greenhome.com

Shower Heads-Chlorine Removing
At EPS, GAI, GEP, HHS.

Silk Quilts
Mulberry Silk: www.silkbedding.com, 1-888-683-8882 or from WYN Enterprises,
1-888-599-6368

Skin Care, Natural
NFS, EPS, www.muskokanaturals.com, or Beebalm & Basil.

The Soap Factory
Unscented hand, dish, laundry & hair products. At NFS & EPS, or contact The Soap Factory 1-800-465-1808.

Tea Tree Oil
At NFS, EPS, & some pharmacies.

Toothpaste, non-fluoridated
At NFS, EPS and some GS.

Udo's Choice Nutrient Products
Digestive enzymes, nutrient powders, Beyond Greens, and oils high in essential fatty acids. At NFS, & some GS. www.fatsthatheal.com Or contact Flora Inc. (see Flora listing above)

Water Pure & Simple—home delivery of reverse osmosis water (8-step processing with ultra violet light & ozone injection) Toronto: 416-721-9689; Vancouver: 604-533-5053

Wobenzym N
Systemic oral enzymes: www.mistergreengenes.com, 702-450-2100

Wood Sealer, low odor
Check at paint and hardware stores. Least toxic version from EPS, HHS, or order Crystal Aire and Crystal Shield Wood Sealers from: Smith's Pharmacy, 416-488-2600 or www.greenhome.com
For similar products check pp. 245-8 in *The Natural House Catalog*.

Wool-stuffed pillows, quilts & baby bunting bags
The Heirloom Wool Company, 204-355-4609, fax 204-355-4919, e-mail: gpries@compuserve.com

Zeolite-Odor-Absorbing Mineral
At EPS, GEP, and HHS.

Cookbooks

Alternative grain recipes; sugar-, dairy-, and wheat-free recipes. Look for these books in libraries, bookstores or NFS, ask your bookstore to order, or order directly from publishers as listed.

The All Natural Allergy Cookbook
Jeanne Marie Martin
Harbour Publishing, P.O. Box 219, Madeira Park, BC, Canada, V0N 2H0

Breaking the Vicious Cycle
Elaine Gottschall
The Kirkton Press, 396 Grills Road, R.R. #2, Baltimore, Ontario, K0K 1C0

The Feel Good Food Guide
Deborah Page Johnson
NewPage Productions, Naperville, IL. Phone: 1-888-468-5800
Includes stevia recipes.

The Self-Healing Cookbook
Kristina Turner
Earthtones Press, P.O. Box 2341-B, Grass Valley, California 95945

The Sugarless Baking Book
Patricia Terris Mayo
Shambala Publications Inc., 1920 13th Street, Boulder, Colorado 80302

Vegetarian Cooking for Everyone
Deborah Madison
Broadway Books, div. of Bantam Doubleday Dell, New York, 1997
(not sugar-free)

Useful Books

Breaking the Vicious Cycle–Intestinal Health Through Diet
Elaine Gottschall, B.A., M.Sc.
The Kirkton Press, Baltimore, Ontario, 1998
Explains how problem foods affect digestion, bowel and brain function, and provides a simple dietary solution including 70 pages of recipes. This diet has helped people with Crohn's disease, colitis, chronic diarrhea, diverticulitis, ordinary indigestion and fatigue.

The Complete Book of Dental Remedies
Flora Parsa Stay, D.D.S.
Avery Publishing Group, Garden City, N.Y., 1996
This book is the *only* book I have seen describing dental conditions and treatments for readers, like me, who did not attend dental school! An excellent reference book if you want to know what's going on in your mouth when you go to the dentist.

Fats that Heal Fats that Kill
Udo Erasmus, Ph.D.
Alive Books, Burnaby, B.C., 1994
This is *the* text on fats and oils, the good and the bad, and how they affect the body in terms of aging, degenerative disease, and chronic conditions. Explains typical (toxic) oil processing and why fats have such a bad reputation. Fascinating, densely-packed information. If you think edible fats and oils only affect body weight, you will learn how important they are to *every* aspect of health!

Food and Healing
Annemarie Colbin
Ballantine, New York, 1996
This is the most complete book I have read on how food affects the human body and mind. Rather than advocating any one style of eating or diet plan, Ms. Colbin explains how many different foods and combinations of foods work to create physical and emotional effects. If you want to understand in detail how to use food to enhance your health and balance your moods this is the book to own.

Healthy Bones
Nancy Appleton, Ph.D.
Avery Publishing Group, Garden City, N.Y., 1991
A straightforward, easy-to-read book about balancing body chemistry to enhance health and prevent osteoporosis. Lots of good info about calcium and how to maintain correct amounts in the body.

The Impossible Child
Doris J. Rapp, M.D.
Practical Allergy Research Foundation, Buffalo, N.Y., 1986
A must-read for parents and teachers. Explains how to recognize if your child has food, chemical or other sensitivities and what to do about them. Dr. Rapp has worked for years

to educate her peers and the public to understand that these sensitivities are real physical afflictions, not psychological imaginings. Clear information and a problem-solving approach.

It's All In Your Head–The Link Between Mercury Amalgams and Illness
Hal Huggins, D.D.S.
Avery Publishing Group, Garden City Park, N.Y., 1993
All the information you need to determine if mercury amalgam fillings may be affecting your health and what to do about them. A little scary, but an invaluable resource for anyone with long-term health problems that don't respond to other treatment.

The Natural House Book Catalog
David Pearson
Fireside, New York, N.Y., 1996
A wonderful source book listing suppliers, products and resources for the home—healthy housewares, bedding, building and renovation materials, air filters, cleaners, furniture, carpets, and more. A must for anyone planning a renovation or new building project.

Nutrition Almanac
John and Gayla Kirschmann
McGraw Hill, New York, N.Y., 1996
A sourcebook listing over 100 ailments and the nutrients that may help correct them. Describes nutrients and herbs, vitamins and minerals that function well together and gives tables of nutritional content of foods. This book works well with *Prescription for Nutritional Healing* to provide a broad spectrum of information.

Potatoes not Prozac
Kathleen DesMaisons, Ph.D.
Simon & Schuster, New York, N.Y., 1998
An important book for anyone who has trouble controlling their blood sugar, experiences roller coaster emotions or uses food or other substances compulsively. DesMaisons shows how brain chemistry affects and is affected by food choices and other activities. Easy to read and packed with useful information. Very important for understanding and coping with addictions of any kind.

The Power of Superfoods
Sam Graci
Prentice Hall, Scarborough, Ont., 1997
Anyone who is ready to move into high-level wellness will want this book. Explains antioxidants, phytonutrients, green drinks, acid/alkaline balance, correct weight loss, as well as a 20-step program for a long, healthy life. Recipe section.

Prescription for Nutritional Healing
James F. Balch, M.D. and Phyllis A. Balch, C.N.C.
Avery Publishing Group, Garden City, N.Y., 1997

This is a must-own reference book for every household. Describes symptoms and possible causes of over 200 disorders, with nutritional and other natural recommendations for healing them. There are clear explanations of the content, actions and uses of herbs, vitamins, minerals, supplements, and other nutrients, and of a variety of remedies and therapies (Color Therapy, Hair Analysis, how to make and use a poultice, etc.)

Sugar Blues
William Dufty
Warner Books, New York, N.Y., 1993
Sugar Blues has been continuously in print since 1975. It is still the number one book about sugar, its history, and its effects on the human body and mind. If you're not afraid to read it, it can change your health permanently for the better.

Take Off Your Glasses and See
Jacob Liberman, O.D., Ph.D.
Crown Trade, New York, N.Y., 1995
How to see more clearly without glasses. Dr. Liberman explains the relationship between eyesight and emotional stress and gives techniques for improving vision naturally (without prescriptive lenses). An extraordinary book that will change your concept of how the eyes work and the possibilities of healing.

What Your Doctor May Not *Tell You About Premenopause*
John R. Lee, M.D.
Warner Books, New York, N.Y., 1999
This is *the* book on hormones and xenohormones. Explains the effects of toxins on the fertility of both sexes. Discusses premenopausal symptoms, what causes them and how to alleviate them. A good source of information on natural progesterone. While this might seem to be a book for women only, parents and parents-to-be will find it invaluable, particularly couples suffering from infertility and parents who wish to protect their children from the genetic consequences of toxic chemicals.

Women's Bodies, Women's Wisdom
Christiane Northrup, M.D.
Bantam Books, New York, N.Y., 1994
Northrup is a physician who got fed up with the medical numbers game and decided to practice in a more holistic way. In this book, she discusses women's health issues not only as a medical doctor focussing on the reproductive cycle from menarche to menopause, but as a woman who values other women's wisdom, emotions, and life experiences as part of what influences their health. Packed with useful and reassuring information.

Index

mutagens, 23, 29, 97, 225
mycotoxins, 11, 93, 227, 231
myopia, 195

N

nail polish, 123, 219
NASA, 83
natural fibers, 42, 44, 48, 97
naturopath, 38, 145
nervousness, 24
nervous system, 9, 17, 18, 35, 36, 41, 67, 106, 145
neurological disease, 106
neurotoxins, 11, 15, 17, 94, 150, 225
neurotransmitters, 64, 133, 196, 197
nicotine, 214
nitrogen, in fertilizer, 116, 117, 120
nitrogen dioxide, & asthma, 54, 88, 213, 228
norepinephrine, 64, 227
nut butter, 137, 138, 155, 156, 160, 163
nutrients, 6, 8, 9, 11, 14, 23, 26, 33, 36, 42, 51, 116, 120, 121, 132, 133, 135, 136, 137, 141, 149, 155, 156, 158, 160, 161, 163, 165, 166, 167, 169, 175, 176, 177, 179, 181, 182, 185, 193, 194, 197, 201, 208, 212, 220, 221, 244, 245
nutritional supplements, 182, 183, 212
nuts, 3, 54, 55, 133, 135, 136, 137, 138, 155, 160, 163, 177, 187, 191, 203, 204, 211

O

obesity, 83, 177, 195, 200
oil lamps, 89
Olbas oil & pastilles, 52, 53, 240
olive oil, 19, 29, 34, 73, 157, 158, 165, 167, 168, 211, 221
oranges, 10, 43, 135, 151
organically-grown food, 60, 63, 108, 125, 135, 136, 141, 142, 143, 156, 173, 183, 189, 202, 203, 204, 211, 222, 229
Ornish, Dean, M.D., 56, 232
osteomalacia, 32, 177, 225
osteoporosis, 32, 175, 176, 177, 178, 179, 180, 181, 213, 223, 225, 230, 244
outgassing, 49, 59, 70, 76, 77, 78, 80, 81, 86, 87, 89, 90, 91, 94, 95, 97, 98, 124
oven cleaner, 67
ovulation, 63
oxalic acid, 173, 177
oxygen, 6, 39, 46, 53, 54, 88, 163, 166, 167, 220

P

paint, 21, 28, 59, 81, 86, 87, 88, 91, 99, 100, 101, 102, 123, 227, 241, 242
Panati, Charles, 23, 35, 225, 226, 227, 232
pancreas, 195, 198, 199, 202, 203
paper towel, 20, 77, 205
paraffin, 16, 27, 29, 58, 89, 124
parasites, 62
particle board, 59, 95, 101, 124
pathways of elimination , 63, 180

pesticides, 10, 33, 48, 63, 94, 96, 99, 105, 106, 107, 108, 109, 116, 119, 120, 123, 130, 135, 141, 142, 143, 145, 156, 159, 163, 168, 181, 202, 218, 222
pest management, 109
petrochemical industry, 15, 29
pets, protecting from toxins, 33, 60, 66, 68, 74, 82, 92, 96, 100, 101, 102, 107, 108, 109, 112, 133, 120, 240
phosphorus, 117, 176, 181, 182
plants & mold, 82, 83, 84, 93, 148, 227
plants & pollution, 82
plastic wrap, 75, 77, 78, 124, 205
plastics & xeno-estrogens, 78
plywood, 95, 98, 101
pneumonia, 50, 226
pollen, 10, 36, 49, 54, 100, 146
pollination, 109
Pomeranz, Bruce, M.D., 50, 226, 233
pot pourri, 58, 85, 91
power lines, 104
pregnancy, 23, 29, 168
preservatives, 19, 133, 135, 156, 160, 209, 234
pressure-treated wood, 102
prunes, 62, 182, 191
psychological disorders, 37

Q

quilts, 124, 241, 242

R

radiant floor heating, 95
radiation, 10, 103, 104, 128, 141, 222
rage, 7, 11, 86, 87
raisins, 132, 156, 160, 191
Randolph, Theron, M.D., 194, 233
Rapp, Doris, M.D., 10, 83, 145, 150, 180, 185, 187, 225, 227, 229, 233, 244
RayAway, 104
Rea, William J., M.D., 15, 226, 227, 233
Reeve, Christopher, 217
reflexology, 152
resins, 36, 99
rice protein powder, 155, 241
rickets, 177
Robertson, Joel, M.D., 55, 64, 196, 197, 222, 227, 233
rotation diet, 137, 138

S

salmonella, 71, 73
salt, 16, 46, 47, 73, 128, 131, 133, 153, 156, 158, 160, 178, 179, 190, 206
sauna, & toxin release, 16, 29, 153
Schweitzer, David, M.D., 195
sea vegetables *see dulse, kelp*
sealers, 86, 101, 242
Seasonal Affective Disorder (SAD), 32, 223
Selye, Hans, 11, 216
serotonin, 55, 60
sesame oil, 33, 225
shoes, 49, 73, 75, 79, 95

We'd love to hear from you!

Questions, comments, feedback, suggestions?
Contact us at:
mail@karenandkathy.com

Or in care of:
Artemis House
Box 1449
Barrie, Ontario
Canada L4M 5R4

Check out our website at:
www.karenandkathy.com

How to Stay Healthy and still Eat Chocolate
makes a great gift!

We will ship books directly to your friends, relatives, or business associates for a special occasion or thank you gift! Just send us their names and addresses with your order. If you include a personal note or card, we will add it to their package.

For bulk orders and quantity discounts, call: 705-792-1898

This book is printed on recyclable paper with vegetable-based inks.

Need more copies of this book? Just fill out the mail order coupon below and mail it, with your payment, to **Artemis House, Box 1449, Barrie, Ontario, L4M 5R4.** For information on workshops or quantity discounts, call us at 705-792-1898. **Order on-line at www.healthyhomeservices.ca.**

✂️- -

Mail Order Coupon

Please send me _____ copies of *How to Stay Healthy and still Eat*

Chocolate @ $24.95 Cdn or $17.95 US each $ _____

Shipping:

N. America: $3.00 for 1 book, $1.00 each additional book $ _____

International: $9.00 first book, $5.00 each additional book $ _____

Canadian residents add 7% GST $ _____

Total enclosed $ _____

Please make cheques or money orders payable to 'Artemis House'.

I have enclosed my ☐ cheque ☐ money order

Please charge my ☐ Visa ☐ Mastercard

Card # _____ Expires _____ / _____

Cardholder name _____

Signature _____

Name: _____

Address: _____

City: _____ Prov./State: _____

P.Code/Zip: _____ Telephone: (____) _____

Email: _____